Sept 17/15

Jill:

Happy
                    Smiles,
Happy Healthy
                    Lives,
Millions of Smiles,
Until 120+ Years.
Bright Blessings,
          Dave.
For the very best!

PRAISE FOR **YOUR MOUTH: THE GATEWAY TO A HEALTHIER YOU**

"Dr. Dana Colson has created a Masterpiece. It will be superbly valued by dental professionals and people from all walks of life who place a high value on oral health."

O. A. Bud Ham, Dental Consultant and Life Coach

"Dana Colson is the kind of dentist you want to open your mouth for, because you feel she cares about you. In this book she will heal your mouth, and your spirit."

Carl Hammerschlag M.D., CPAE, Yale-trained psychiatrist, University of Arizona Medical School faculty member
Author, *The Dancing Healers, The Theft of the Spirit* and *Healing Ceremonies*

"This book about modern whole-person dentistry is enjoyable to read and easy-to-grasp. It contains many insights and practical ideas, not just about mouth health but about taking care of the Whole You!"

Lynn M. Marshall M.D., FAAEM, FRSM, MCFP
Faculty of Medicine, University of Toronto, Lakehead and Laurentian Universities
President and Chair of the Board, Environmental Health Institute of Canada
Medical Education Liaison/Staff Physician, Environmental Health Clinic

"In this entertaining and well-written book, Dr. Dana Colson presents the reader with a clear picture of how the mouth is a guide to general health. Using a combination of recent scientific advances and intriguing glimpses into the past, Y*our Mouth: The Gateway to a Healthier You* provides many practical tips on maintaining good oral care and supporting better general health. Dr. Colson's book is an excellent place to start understanding the emerging new paradigm for dentistry."

Gavin James, Orthodontist, B.D.S., M.D.S., F.D.S. (Eng), D. Orthodontics

"In her book *Your Mouth: The Gateway to a Healthier You*, Dana Colson takes us on a journey that masterfully links the seemingly disjointed parts of the physical body to their relationship in our mouths. In essence, Dana is a visionary who is able to articulate the dental connections of the mind, body and spirit."

Catherine Hornby, Doctor of Chiropractic Medicine, B.Sc.N,
Acupuncturist and Craniosacral Therapist

"I highly recommend *Your Mouth: The Gateway to a Healthier You* not only for dental and other healthcare practitioners, but also for each of us and all those we love and care about, as a powerful tool for achieving a rich understanding of the place of the mouth in our own overall health."

Wilson Southam, Past President, The Group at Cox
and Co-author, *The Spirit of Volitional Practice*

"*Your Mouth: The Gateway to a Healthier You* is an essential, accessible and entertaining read for anyone seeking a simple and direct path to a healthier, happier and more confident daily life. Honestly, the only thing I would do to improve it would be make it longer! It left me wanting more!"

Christopher Heard, Author, TV and radio personality and
very grateful patient!

"Since reading Dana's book, I am able to enjoy my mouth yoga whenever I need it, using *'lips together, teeth apart, and tongue in place.'* This simple meditative exercise provides not only instant tension relief for my jaw, but it also relieves any tension I have in my head and neck as well. Thanks, Dana!"

Emily Ridout, Co-founder of 889 Yonge - Yoga + Wellness Spa

The techniques, ideas and suggestions in this book are being provided for informational purposes only and are not intended as a substitute for proper medical and/or dental advice, diagnosis or treatment. Always consult your physician, dentist or healthcare professional with any questions you may have regarding a medical and/or dental condition and before performing any new exercise technique or beginning any new diet. Neither the publisher nor the author of this book make any warranty of any kind in regard to its content.

The content of this book is accurate as of the date of publication; however, as new information and products become available, some of the content may become invalid. You should always seek the most up-to-date information from your healthcare practitioner. Neither the publisher nor the author of this book shall be liable or responsible to any person or entity for any errors contained in this book, or for any special, incidental or consequential damage caused or alleged to be caused directly or indirectly by the information contained within.

YOUR MOUTH: THE GATEWAY TO A HEALTHIER YOU

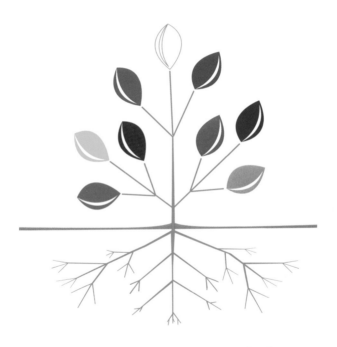

A yoga-based approach to exploring the connections between oral health, whole body wellness and longevity.

Dana G. Colson, D.D.S.

© Copyright 2011 Dana G. Colson D.D.S.

All rights reserved. No part of this book may be reproduced or transmitted in any form by any means, electronic or mechanical, including photocopying, recording, or by any information storage and retrieval system without the prior written permission of the author, except for the inclusion of brief quotations in critical reviews and certain other noncommercial uses permitted by copyright law. For permission requests, please contact the author in writing at the address below.

FIRST EDITION

Library and Archives Canada Cataloguing in Publication

Colson, Dana G.
    Your mouth : the gateway to a healthier you : a yoga-based approach to exploring the connections between oral health, whole body wellness and longevity / Dana G. Colson.

Includes bibliographical references and index.
ISBN 978-0-9869370-0-2

1. Mouth--Care and hygiene. 2. Health.
3. Longevity. 4. Yoga. I. Title.

RA776.C63 2011
613   C2011-903188-4

Published by DJC Corp.
1950 Yonge Street, Toronto, Ontario, Canada M4S 1Z4

This book is available at special quantity discounts for educational, business or promotional use. Please visit www.yourmouththegatewaytoahealthieryou.com for pricing and ordering information.

Printed in Canada

MIX
Paper from
responsible sources
FSC FSC® C016245

This book is dedicated to my patients and everyone else who has impacted me on my journey.

And to Jeffrey and Caitlin: my fabulous children who continue to seek and quest and love life... may it continue to be a passionate journey.

TABLE OF CONTENTS

A MESSAGE FROM THE AUTHOR

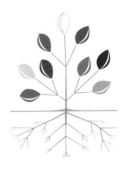

The mouth is one of the body's most powerful instruments. Without it, we couldn't survive. It is how we get our nutrition and satisfy our thirst.

It's the means by which we communicate and articulate our thoughts and feelings—how we share ourselves with our friends, our neighbors and our communities. It is also a lighthouse for the human spirit. When we smile, we radiate light and impart our energy.

As a dentist, I believe it is important to communicate with those entrusted to my care. My philosophy has always been one of empowering my patients with education. I know that when patients open their mouths, they are giving me their trust. It is impossible to underestimate the importance of building trust through active listening. I've come to realize that, in many ways, my patients are often their own best physicians. Listening gives me a deeper understanding and awareness of what they are truly experiencing. Then following through with a clinical examination gives me a much clearer picture of the best course of treatment.

It is a two-way communication that creates the most favorable outcome.

I have been practicing dentistry for more than 30 years. I never feel like I go to work. My work is who I am and what I do; it's my passion, my hobby and my life. In some ways it's remarkable that I made this career choice, given the confession I am about to make: growing up I hated going to the dentist. The dentist terrified me. To help get me through my appointments, my mother always promised that I could go to the toy store and pick out a game or puzzle if I would just sit quietly and let the dentist do his work. Luckily, I sailed through my teenage years without a single cavity.

Then, one day, a chance meeting on the bus while traveling to my home town of Peterborough, Ontario, proved fortuitous. I ran into an acquaintance from my neighborhood. We were the same age and both in undergraduate programs at university. He asked me what I was planning to study. At the time I had been thinking very seriously about medicine. He told me that he was going to study dentistry. He had just returned from an open house at the University of Toronto, where he discovered that dentists worked with laughing gas and that there were all kinds of toothbrushes–not just the kind we bought at the drugstore. I was riveted. Perhaps, if I could become a dentist, I could help *other* people overcome their fear of going to the dentist.

My fascination was further piqued in dental school with the first lecture on the mouth-body connection. Some of the pictures my professors used in their lectures were, quite frankly, shocking. I'd never seen an image on a large screen of a mouth pulled open so wide–showing not just the teeth, but the gum tissue and tongue. Sometimes the mouth was healthy. But often the pictures showed decay and various states of disease. Those images stayed with me. In fact, they became part of my lifelong quest to understand how the body mirrors itself in the mouth and vice versa.

I've always been committed to keeping up on the latest scientific advancements. I have continued my education each and every year through seminars and professional development. And I have always sought to share this knowledge with my patients.

I believe mine is an approach that corresponds with many of the same values and principles found in the practice of yoga. Yoga is about expansion and opening ourselves up to a higher power. It is fundamentally about empowerment. Ultimately, I live to work *with* my patients rather than *on* them. I aim to give them an opportunity to participate in their treatment plan and healing.

Some would argue that the Golden Age of Dentistry has passed because we have now figured out how to help people preserve their teeth over a lifetime. However, I believe we're entering the most exciting period in dentistry yet. Not only have dentists' responsibilities expanded as we take on a larger role in protecting our patients against the threat of serious illness, but technology has given us the tools to create spectacular smiles. I believe that people ought to be able to keep their teeth until they are 120. But even if you live to be 80 or 90, wouldn't it be great to say you had the best smile until the last day of your life? What other part of the body can we say is going to be the very best until the end?

In the spirit of empowerment, continuous education and imparting knowledge, I would like to share my passion and what I have learned in more than three decades of practice. If you have an amazing smile, celebrate and treasure it. And if you have a friend or loved one who doesn't, please share this book with them. That's what friends and family do—support and celebrate each other through the journey and school of life. If this book empowers just one person, and helps them release their fear as I was able to do, then it has succeeded.

Dana G. Colson, D.D.S.

1

THE POWER OF THE MOUTH

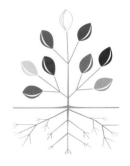

Our mouth is, first and foremost, the means by which we take in our nutrients and where digestion begins.

It plays a social and sexual role—we kiss those we love. The mouth also plays a primary role in the way we communicate. Our voice, for example, is produced in the throat, while the tongue, lips, teeth and jaws are all needed to produce the range of sounds that make up our speech.

You might even say that our words determine our destiny. According to psychologists, optimistic words lead to happiness—both for the person thinking and speaking positively, and for the listener. This contributes to the success of our relationships, our work lives and even our company's bottom line.

Our mouth is a part of how we make the sounds of laughter and, of course, how we smile. Our smile plays a major role in how we perceive ourselves and others. Just as a radiant smile opens the world up to us and reflects positive energy, an unattractive smile holds us back. When we don't like the aesthetics of our mouth, it is more difficult to speak our truths, to be authentic and to embrace the world.

Our response to aesthetics seems to be hardwired. We know that babies respond to faces that are more attractive. Good-looking men and women get better and more prestigious jobs. A 2004 study by the American Academy of Cosmetic Dentistry shows that 99 percent of those surveyed believe that an attractive smile is an important social asset, while 96 percent believe that an attractive smile makes a person more appealing to the opposite sex. Meanwhile, 74 percent feel a bad smile can ruin your chance of career success.

Teeth in Times Past

We have always viewed our teeth as something more than just tools for chewing and shredding food. Long before whitening strips, braces and porcelain veneers, primitive people sought to enhance their appearance with beautiful teeth. The Mayans filled their teeth with colorful inlays of jade and gold. Young girls in the Ticuna tribe of Brazil traditionally filed their teeth into sharp points as a mark of beauty. On the other side of the world,

Hindus in Bali file their teeth to symbolically remove aggressive behavior and mark the passage from puberty to adulthood in a ceremony that takes place prior to their wedding day.

Even cavemen were obsessed with preserving their teeth. In 2001, archaeologists digging at a Neolithic gravesite in Pakistan, estimated to be between 7,000 and 9,000 years old, uncovered evidence of humankind's earliest dentistry. They found half a dozen molars that had been drilled with flint heads, revealing a complex procedure in which the tooth's cavity wall was carved out to remove decay. Researchers believe that these early dentists were probably the tribe's bead workers, whose skills also proved useful in fixing teeth.

Early in their history even the ancient Greeks hadn't achieved this degree of sophistication. They initially believed that tooth decay was caused by spirits. They sought cures for toothaches and decay through magic and prayer. Not until the arrival of Hippocrates (BC 460-376), the father of modern medicine, were those notions dispelled. Hippocrates sought scientific evidence and set out to separate medicine from religion. He posited that disease wasn't a punishment inflicted by the gods, but the product of diet and lifestyle.

In his journals, Hippocrates wrote extensively about problems with the teeth and gums, raising possible connections between what happened in the oral cavity and the rest of the body. He believed that tooth decay was caused by the corrosive action of food, in addition to individual predisposition. He also invented a number of dental instruments, including forceps for extraction, and advocated cleaning the teeth with small wooden sticks and wool moistened with honey.

Based on Hippocrates' early work, the glory of Rome was said to be reflected in the mouths of its most prominent citizens. Clean teeth were so valued by affluent families that they had their slaves clean their mouths daily. Poets and writers of the time also celebrated teeth as a fundamental aspect of a woman's beauty and an orator's diction.

Reading Smiles

What makes a beautiful smile? In many ways, the basics of a great smile mirror the principles of yoga. A beautiful smile radiates vitality. Like yoga, it's about proper alignment. And it doesn't just look good, it functions well too. A healthy mouth depends on the shape of each tooth in relation to the others, its alignment, its bite and its position relative to the lips and tongue.

We can also read faces for clues to other kinds of health issues that originate in the oral cavity. A weak chin with a bite misalignment, for example, may contribute to low oxygen intake, headache or neck pain. The telltale signs of sleep apnea–a disruption of breathing during sleep–are often clearly visible on the face.

It's a happy coincidence that well-functioning teeth and good-looking teeth are so intimately connected. When we achieve the best smile we possibly can, it changes our lives, making us more social and increasing the release of endorphins which helps our immune system. Just as yoga tones our body, smiling tones and exercises our facial muscles. And a toned face looks younger! After all, beautiful teeth make us want to smile, and smiling is our best natural vitamin.

Age Reversal Through Dentistry

While research shows that attractive smiles boost

our performance in both the boardroom and the boudoir, a beautiful smile has another powerful advantage: it can take years off the face. A wide, white and beautiful smile radiates youth, while cracked, stained or chipped teeth can make us look much older than we really are.

The two upper and lower cuspids (canines) are our longest teeth, with long, firmly implanted roots, and provide an actual framework for our smile. The fullness of our lips and mouth is wrapped over these long teeth. If we grind our teeth to the point where they are broken, flattened or severely worn, we end up with sagging skin around our mouths, resulting in a much older appearance.

The vast majority of facial aging occurs in the lower third of the face. Even if we look at the face of someone in his or her mid-20s, the early signs of aging are already setting in. These visible changes include:

- descent of the eyebrows
- descent of the nasal tip
- descent of the chin tip
- sinking of the nasal bone.

Signs of aging visible in the mouth are evident when:

- teeth become crowded
- teeth wear down
- tooth shape and proportion changes
- tooth color changes
- changes occur to soft tissue.

A decrease in collagen and elastin also causes a laxness and thinning of the skin, leading to dramatic changes in the lips and the entire oral complex.

In younger faces, two to three millimeters of the teeth are visible when the lips are relaxed. As we get older, through grinding, clenching and other wear and tear, we tend to have less "vertical dimension"–that is, our teeth become shorter. By restoring teeth and preventing further grinding and clenching, we bring back the youthful look of our teeth. Expanding the arch formation of teeth through orthodontics is like augmenting the scaffolding, allowing for better draping of the soft tissues. What's more, a wider smile adds volume and props up the upper lip, thus helping to smooth the wrinkles above the lips and contributing to a younger appearance.

New Directions

Dentistry has undoubtedly evolved more quickly in the past two decades than ever before. While technology has given practitioners powerful new tools, science has provided a new understanding of both health and aesthetics. But there is also something larger at play: social attitudes toward dentistry are changing. It is no longer something to be afraid of–with new technology and new approaches, the opportunity to take care of our mouths is something to be embraced.

Minimally invasive dentistry is now possible due to advances in technology and materials. Dentists are looking for the simplest, least-invasive ways to correct dental problems. Whether it's fixing cavities, treating periodontal disease or creating a more beautiful smile, the philosophy is based on three ideals: identify, prevent and restore. The goal is always to perform the least amount of dentistry to restore the teeth and gums to health.

Oral health is now being regarded in the context of whole body health. Many colleges and universities across North America are already revamping their curricula to reflect this change. The dental practitioner is seen not only as someone who attends to cavities and creates beautiful smiles, but as part of a team of multidisciplinary healthcare providers unified in working toward the goal of reducing and preventing chronic disease.

Dental teams take our blood pressures and health histories, and, increasingly, gather insights about risk factors impacting our oral health. They take down histories of tobacco use and soft drink consumption, record information about diet, observe neck size and note activity levels. Ultimately, they view all of this information to screen for any health alerts. Their role is primarily one of referral–helping to prevent conditions like heart disease and diabetes by referring patients for more in-depth evaluations if risk factors are evident.

Dentists are also increasingly called upon to be the gatekeepers, the first line of defense to ensure our overall health and wellness. By creating a healthier mouth, we pave the way for a healthier body. The goal is to encourage a stress-free mouth in order to ensure a stress-free body. As practitioners of yoga teach us how to be more mindful of our body, dentists teach us to care for and respect the mouth. Both are journeys with better health as the final destination. Our quality of daily and professional care, combined with our awareness, leads to healthier teeth and gum tissue that will serve us over a lifetime.

As we move forward, the role of the dental practitioner will expand and physicians, nurses, pharmacists, dentists, dental hygienists and other healthcare practitioners will continue to work together to increase communication, demystify the mouth and how it affects the rest of the body and empower the dental team.

Making the Connections

We have long known that there is a close connection between health in the mouth and health in the rest of the body. But over the past decades science has unraveled a number of previously unknown connections–links between our oral health and heart disease, diabetes, obesity and even pregnancy complications.

The role of the dentist has changed in some crucial ways. Increasingly, it's their job not only to create amazing smiles, but also to be the gatekeepers in identifying and hopefully minimizing other diseases. Dentists can impart to patients the power of smiling, which triggers an endorphin boost, stabilizing blood pressure, relaxing muscles, improving respiration and speeding up healing.

The Report on Oral Health in America (2000) concluded that oral health and general health are inseparable and that oral health is integral to general health. It recognized the mouth as a portal of entry for infections that can spread to other parts of the body and acknowledged a need to change non-dental healthcare providers' perception of the importance of oral health.

Armed with the knowledge provided in this book, we can recognize and take responsibility for our choices and create healthy mouths and bodies, allowing us to experience and enjoy life to its fullest!

The Power of the Mouth

2

THE WHOLE BODY CONNECTION

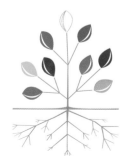

The year was 1840–a pivotal time for dentistry and human health in general.

Two enterprising dental health practitioners, Drs. Horace Hayden and Chapin Harris, founded the world's first dental college at the University of Maryland. Until the establishment of this school, oral health fell within the domain of two very different sorts of practitioners. On the one hand, barbers or tradesman pulled rotting teeth and helped fashion dental appliances like bridges and dentures. On the other, elite practitioners specialized in dentistry.

The establishment of the Western world's first professional dental school united these disparate disciplines; however, it was a mixed blessing. While it was a positive development in many ways, it meant that dental and medical schools would become separate faculties. More recently, study upon study is finding that the health of our body has an impact on the health of our mouth and vice versa.

Scientists are only just beginning to understand the role of inflammation in whole body health.

They are gradually gaining a better appreciation, for instance, of the links between periodontal disease and other serious health issues, such as diabetes, cardiovascular disease and pregnancy complications, including miscarriages and premature births. Physicians agree that patients who have undergone organ transplants or other major medical interventions have a greater chance for successful recovery if they maintain good oral health before and after their operation. Good oral health has also been cited as one of the conditions for a longer life–adding as much as 6.4 years!

Former U.S. Surgeon General
Dr. David Satcher called gum
disease "the silent epidemic"
in his 2000 report.

What Is Periodontal (Gum) Disease?

Periodontal or gum disease is an inflammatory process that affects the tissues that support and anchor the teeth. The progression of gum disease is episodic and requires constant supervision. There are a wide range of symptoms. Some are subtle and, in the early stage (gingivitis), might not be readily noticed: redness; bleeding and irritation of gums when brushing, flossing or even biting; and bad breath. The symptoms of a more advanced state (periodontitis) affect the gum and bone. They are more obvious: the apparent lengthening or shifting of teeth (a process that spawned the phrase "long in the tooth" in 19th century England); the perception of loose teeth; and, in the most severe cases, abscesses and infections. If left untreated, teeth can fall out or may have to be removed.

There can be as many bacteria in the human mouth as there are cells in the body. Over 500 species have been identified. Gum disease is caused by bacteria that reside in the plaque that builds up between teeth and the gingiva (the gum tissue around the tooth). As the plaque hardens

The growing list of risk factors for periodontal disease:

- Smoking (the number one risk factor)
- Diabetes
- Genetics
- Age
- Stress
- Lower income and less education
- Inactivity
- Osteoporosis
- Immune disorders
- Hormonal influences
- H. pylori infections
- Contact with others' saliva
- Dietary deficiencies
- Chronic kidney disease
- HIV
- Use of some prescription medications

and becomes calculus, also known as tartar, it sticks to teeth along and just below the gum line.

When the plaque calcifies above and below the gum tissue, the calculus cannot be removed by simple brushing. The size of the gum pocket increases, allowing the bacterial plaque to flourish. More advanced strains of plaque can cause serious infections, resulting in the loss of tooth-supporting tissue, including bone. This can alter pathways in the immune system that may be harmful to other systems in the body.

Note that since the majority of oral bacteria flourishes on the tongue surface, it is also important for us to clean our tongues regularly.

The Role of Inflammation in Disease

In 1998, the American Academy of Periodontology began serious efforts to educate society on the connection between inflammation in the mouth and overall health, stating that "infection in the mouth can play havoc elsewhere in the body." Scientists estimate that two-thirds of the damage from periodontitis is caused by inflammation, the body's response to the bacteria,

Certain ethnicities are more genetically predisposed to gum disease, including Asians, Hispanics and African Americans.

rather than the bacterial infection itself. Inflammation is the way our body's immune system thwarts an invasive attack, but when inflammation becomes chronic, or the pathways triggered by inflammation are not "switched off," it can do a great deal of damage to the body.

If gingivitis and periodontitis go undetected or untreated and the bacterial infection escalates, the immune system's reaction escalates as well. Bacteria-fighting white blood cells respond, congregating at the site of gum damage and engulfing the bacteria. Inflammation results. Unfortunately, the white blood cells, or the defense pathways triggered by their actions, kill not only bacteria, but anything else that strays into their line of fire. Irreversible gum disease and underlying bone loss will then inevitably occur, which could lead to tooth loss.

There is also a clear genetic disposition for gum disease and the prevalence of this disease varies within different populations.

It is the potential damage to various systems of the body that makes the diagnosis and treatment of gum disease an ongoing and life-altering endeavor.

Diabetes is a chronic, lifelong illness. Approximately 6.8% of the population has been diagnosed with diabetes, while another 20% is considered "pre-diabetic," or on the verge of developing diabetes. It is projected that the number of people with diabetes will increase to 8.9% by 2020.

Gum Disease and Diabetes

Over the past decade evidence has been mounting that patients with uncontrolled or poorly controlled diabetes are much more likely to develop gum or periodontal disease, or periodontal disease with greater severity. The converse is also true. Control of diabetes, a rather complex effort under any circumstances, can be a lot easier when periodontal disease is controlled.

Periodontal disease begins with a bacterial infection. As our immune system fights the infection, the activated cells produce inflammatory biological signals (cytokines) that have a destructive effect throughout the entire body. Some cytokines cause insulin resistance and elevated blood-sugar levels that can be a factor in the onset of diabetes.

The good news: studies show that the treatment of periodontal disease has the potential to improve glucose control and reduce insulin requirements.

A study published in 2010 by a UC Berkeley health researcher suggests that women who receive regular dental care reduce their risk of heart attacks, stroke and other cardiovascular problems by at least one-third.

Gum Disease and Heart Disease

In the summer of 2009 researchers teamed up to publish a revised series of recommendations for both medical and dental professionals in managing those at risk for heart or gum disease, or both. It was a clear acknowledgment of one fact: people with periodontal disease are almost twice as likely to suffer from coronary artery disease as those without periodontal disease.

Looking back, even as recently as a decade ago, heart disease was viewed as a rather easily explained plumbing problem. However, a landmark paper published in *The New England Journal of Medicine* in 1999 raised new questions about the cause of cardiovascular disease. Up until that point it was assumed that heart disease was simply a narrowing and blocking of arteries due to a build-up of fatty plaque along the interior walls of the blood vessels. When the arteries were fully blocked, the heart or the brain would be starved of blood, causing a heart attack or stroke. If the plaque broke away, it could cause a blood clot. These catastrophic events were long presumed to be a simple failure of the circulatory

Pregnant women who have periodontal disease may be seven times more likely to have a premature baby. Premature birth can lead to some serious consequences for the baby.

system, physically no more complicated than a blocked drain.

Now research is revealing that atherosclerosis (thickening of the arteries) is much more complex at the cellular level than previously believed. It is more connected to bacterial damage in the lining of the arteries due to the inflammatory process. Increasingly, both dentists and physicians are addressing the total inflammatory burden on the body and how periodontal disease—a low-grade systemic inflammation—interconnects and contributes to systemic diseases. A large body of evidence indicates that systemic (widespread) inflammation is present in patients with periodontal disease and that such inflammation is a risk factor for other diseases as well.

Gum Disease and Pregnancy

There is evidence that oral infection, everything from mild gingivitis to full-blown periodontitis, puts pregnant women at risk for complications, including miscarriages and premature births. Contributing to this is the fact that a change in a pregnant woman's hormones can cause gums to

Basics of Home Dental Care:

- Brush for two minutes in a routine pattern to ensure each tooth has been properly cleaned

- Use a rotary or sonic vibration toothbrush

- Floss daily

- Massage irritated tissue with a specialized tool from your dentist

- If using a mouth rinse, make sure it's nonalcoholic

- Brush your tongue or use a special tongue scraper to remove bacteria

- Maintain a schedule of regular dental visits to maximize the quality of your gum health

Note:

Most bad breath originates from bacteria on the tongue.

Bleeding gums are not normal and can lead to serious health problems.

bleed more vigorously and can also promote the growth of bacteria. In this way bacteria can enter the bloodstream in greater numbers and reach the developing fetus. This condition, when extreme, is known as pregnancy gingivitis.

For this reason more frequent visits with a dental hygienist are important for pregnant women in order to keep their gum tissues healthy.

Mounting Evidence

There's mounting evidence of a cascade of illnesses and diseases associated with gum disease.

Both the professions of medicine and dentistry are increasingly aware of the importance of a healthy mouth, not only to maintain our teeth, but also to contribute to our overall well-being.

3

GRINDING, CLENCHING AND HEADACHES

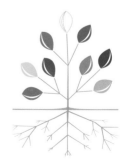

Monitoring jaw and tooth development is crucial to oral health.

Dentistry can create a foundation so that our teeth have the opportunity to form properly without protruding or becoming crowded—consequences that impede the proper support and development of the jaws and may lead to a lifetime of headache pain, among other issues.

When we grind or clench our teeth, we may wear through our enamel, exposing softer tooth structure called dentin. Fracture lines in the enamel may also be created. When the enamel begins to chip and the dentin erodes, the teeth begin to break and flatten. If this occurs on the front teeth, we can wear away so much enamel that our teeth are no longer parallel to our lips, resulting in a "negative smile." Our back teeth will also no longer fit the same way, as we've altered the original anatomy. What once resembled hills and valleys can become flattened or hollowed-out surfaces.

A misalignment, muscle tension or stress can set grinding and clenching into motion, especially during sleep. The gnashing sets off a constant spasm of muscles in the jaws, which can lead to severe tension headaches. Just as yoga makes use of the radiating effects of small movements, even small realignments of the bite can have a dramatic impact on our health.

Positive Smile

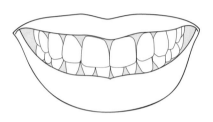

Negative Smile

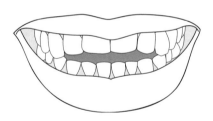

When we grind or clench our teeth, we can wear away so much enamel that our teeth are no longer parallel to our lips, resulting in a "negative smile."

Headaches

In North America today it's considered "normal" to experience headaches. The majority of people experience tension headaches that can be felt around the eyes and ears. Scientists are working to understand the cause rather than just to treat the symptoms. Indeed, medical resources are increasingly devoted to trying to understand the underlying conditions that give rise to headaches.

The message that needs to be delivered to thousands of headache sufferers is that having headaches is not normal. A dentist may ask if one experiences headaches, and diagnose if they are related to jaw position, clenching or grinding.

Here are some signs that a headache may have a dental origin:

- pain or pressure beside the eye
- pain originating behind the eyes
- congestion
- ringing in the ears
- dizziness
- sore neck muscles or tension
- clicking or grating noises in jaw joints

Having headaches is not normal.

- tired jaw muscles
- head or scalp painful to the touch
- pain in cheeks, jaw joints or teeth
- radiating pain in the neck and shoulders, sometimes even the back.

Luckily, there are many ways to reduce or eliminate this pain without drugs or surgery. Less invasive treatments include stress reduction, jaw exercises and trigger-point therapy. If these fail to relieve headaches, a dentist may recommend a bite plate or mouth guard that creates a smooth surface to help prevent the interlocking of tooth surfaces. Eliminating clenching and gnashing prevents the tightening of muscles that restrict blood flow and creates head "aches." These methods will be discussed in more detail later in this section.

Two of the most common dental causes of tension headaches are grinding and clenching, and jaw misalignment.

Grinding and Clenching

Broken, chipped or fractured teeth and receding gums are often signs of grinding and clenching. Some people clench and grind their teeth only

Unsure if you grind and clench your teeth? Here is a checklist of other possible signs:

- Do you get headaches, even slight headaches, especially in the early part of the day?
- Are your headaches located beside or behind your eyes?
- Do you wake up feeling like your teeth have had a workout?
- Do your teeth fit very tightly together in the morning?
- Are your jaw muscles sore in the morning?
- Do you have tenderness in the cheek area, especially beneath the cheek bones and in front of your ears?
- Does your tongue have a ridged or scalloped edge when resting in the mouth?

during sleep. Others clench their teeth during the day, usually when they are tense or anxious. Over time it becomes a lifelong habit–often one of which we're unaware.

It's estimated that about 5 to 6 percent of us grind excessively, yet most of us will suffer bouts of grinding and clenching at some point in our lives. Research shows that it is equally prevalent in both sexes, but more common in younger people.

When we grind or clench we can exert up to or over 550 pounds of pressure per square inch! That's a lot of pressure. The associated noise resembles that of cracking into a hard nut and can wake up our bed partner.

Causes of Grinding and Clenching

The reasons for teeth grinding are complex and varied, but essentially the cause is an imbalance in the body, whether physical or emotional.

When life gets tough, or we're feeling frustration or anger, too often our reaction is to clench or grind our teeth. Bite misalignment is a common physical cause. When our bite is imbalanced, it's

Scalloped Tongue

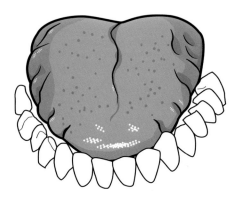

The tongue is an extremely strong muscle. When we clench or grind our teeth, our tongue steps in to brace the jaws, an action that eventually creates telltale signs of pinch marks around the edges. In this way, our tongue gives a dentist important information about the positioning of our jaws. Like the lines on our face after falling asleep on a corduroy couch, the tongue gives us a sign that we are probably clenching our teeth.

natural to grind our teeth involuntarily at night to try to correct the situation or help improve our airway. There may also be a neuromuscular cause. The position of the head can also affect how teeth are aligned. If one holds one's head too far forward, as a result of whiplash, limited airways, genetics or simply bad posture, it can contribute to grinding or clenching.

Much like gum disease, grinding and clenching can be difficult to detect in its initial stages. It is frequently not a recognized habit. Often by the time it is diagnosed, it has advanced, which complicates treatment. Grinding and clenching do not always result in headaches, but can still damage our teeth and jaw joints.

Relief from Grinding and Clenching

We may be able to consciously prevent ourselves from grinding and clenching while we are awake–there are a number of methods that we will discuss beginning on page 53–but it is when we are asleep that we often require help.

There are a variety of dental appliances available to prevent teeth from meshing together and reduce

Like bones, teeth are not meant to touch each other directly when at rest. Think of your vertebrae; if the bones were touching each other you would be in pain.

the pressure on the jaw joint. The use of such appliances–bite plates, deprogrammers, splints and specialized mouth guards–provide remarkable relief. They work by minimizing the assault on the teeth's surface, reducing the tightening of muscles, and sometimes actually deprogramming the muscles. Bite plates also help stabilize the bite by helping to prevent the gradual shifts, crowding and wear that accompany grinding and clenching.

A longer-term solution may involve restructuring the bite to ease the stress on the jaw muscles, thus eliminating the grind and clench response. This may often be achieved with a bite adjustment or orthodontics (such as invisible braces), restorative dentistry, dental surgery or a combination of the above. When exploring the various treatments available, it is important to be aware that, due to the complex nature of the body, even these procedures may not fully resolve symptoms. All noninvasive, reversible treatments should be explored before considering any procedure that may permanently alter tooth arrangement or jaw position.

Diagnosing TMD

Temporomandibular joint (TMJ) syndrome or disorder (TMD) is related to our jaw joints. We have two TMJs, one on each side of our jaws, which connect the lower jaw to the skull in front of the ear. TMJ problems can result in jaws that are locked in position or difficult to open, bite misalignment, as well as ringing in the ears, or head or neck pain.

Your dentist can often diagnose TMD based on a physical examination of your face, your jaws and your muscles. Dentists who treat TMD also use extensive questionnaires and other technologies to find out why you have pain in your jaws, head or neck.

What Are the Jaws?

Jaws are an incredibly clever feat of skeletal engineering. They consist of two jawbones, the upper jawbone, known as the maxilla, and the lower jawbone, called the mandible. The temporomandibular joint (TMJ) connects the mandible to the head at the temporal bone.

The TMJ is located just in front of the ears. It acts like a hinge, allowing us to open and close our mouths and chew from side to side. It works in tandem with a number of muscles and supporting structures. The TMJ is a central element of the head-neck-jaw complex. It contains a piece of cartilage called a disc, which keeps the temporal bone and the jawbone from rubbing against each other. If jaws become overworked or overloaded, this cartilage can become damaged and slip out of position, causing clicks, cracks or popping sounds—or even a locked jaw—when opening or closing.

Our jaws also help us to balance. An adult human head typically weighs between eight and twelve pounds, yet it is balanced with only seven vertebrae in our necks. Balance is maintained by

Radiating Pain

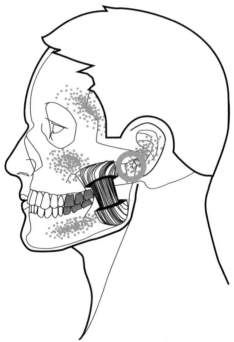

When the masseter muscle is stressed due to teeth clenching together, it can cause pain to radiate—or even be isolated—to other areas of the face and jaw. These areas are indicated by the gray dots in the above illustration.

◯ Location of TMJ

the lower jaw and its muscles, which counterweigh the rest of the skull. When the jaws are sitting properly, they rest comfortably, as do the head and shoulders. But if the lower jaw is out of place, it can throw the jaw muscles out of balance, putting a strain on the neck and head. If our head is tilted as little as eight degrees forward, 35 to 40 pounds of pull is required by the posterior neck muscles to maintain the head in an optimal posture. This kind of strain on the neck muscles can cause pain to radiate to other parts of the body, resulting in neck strain and headaches.

Our teeth are also critically important to well-functioning jaws. They are the pillars that support the entire structure. Although by age 6 most of our head and jaw development is complete, jaw and tooth development actually continue until we are in our mid- to late-20s. If the jaws and teeth don't develop properly, they can contribute to a bite misalignment–called malocclusion. Often, the lower and/or upper jaw can be set either too far back or forward or jaws are mismatched in size. Malocclusion can vary in severity.

Narrow Arches

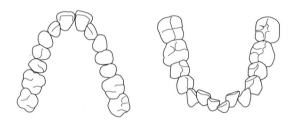

Wide Arches

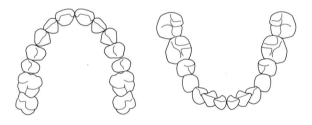

A wider arch allows for proper tongue position, better cleanse ability and better function of teeth.

How Do Our Jaws Become Misaligned?

Various factors can cause jaws to shift, putting strain on the surrounding tissues and muscles in our mouths. If teeth are never formed, or pulled because of fractures, abscesses or unsuccessful root canal therapy, the position of our jaws can be modified when the remaining teeth shift over time due to the loss. Misalignment may also be the result of genetics, environmental factors or mouth breathing–breathing through the mouth rather than through the nose when at rest or during light exercise–which over time can lead to altered tongue position and shifting of the teeth. Mouth breathing is most often due to obstructions or allergies and causes swelling in the tonsils and adenoids. This can persist even after orthodontic treatment and cause relapse. Sometimes bite misalignment can also begin with whiplash, a slight blow to the head or even arthritis.

Jaw problems are also caused by poor oral habits in children. For example, children who suck their thumbs beyond four years of age can push their growing teeth out of position by molding their upper palate with their thumb or fingers, which

Over the centuries we've found ingenious and sometimes dubious ways to dull headache pain. As far back as 5,000 years ago primitive peoples took to drilling holes in the tops of their skulls–a process called trepanation–for relief. Thankfully, by the 13th century headache sufferers discovered less invasive methods, relieving headaches with potions made from opium and vinegar. And while the early Puritans in America believed that headache pain was part of God's plan and must simply be endured, folk remedies flourished in the colonies. Since many believed pain was caused by evil forces, they sought cures that included prayer, incantations and amulets. Others treated their pain with moss gathered from the heads of statues found in the town's squares. And many others commonly sought relief with mustard plasters and baths. By the 19th century, pharmacists began tinkering with the chemicals culled from willow bark to relieve pain and inflammation–thus developing the precursor to Aspirin®.

can create narrow arches, cross-bites and high-vaulted roofs in their mouths. Such conditions also encourage mouth breathing and an open bite, which can lead to more serious issues. Children then swallow, pushing their tongue against teeth that do not meet in order to create a closed space. The tongue is one of our most powerful muscles and the sheer strength of its thrust when swallowing can prevent a child from developing a normal bite. It is also common for children to grind or clench their teeth, putting undue stress on their teeth and jaws. Fortunately, this is a habit that many children leave behind when their permanent teeth come in.

Being Mindful and Developing Good Habits

Just as yoga promotes the melting away of tension and pain through the mindful practice of proper poses, paying attention to proper jaw alignment and doing facial exercises and massage to encourage proper positioning can relieve headache pain and other problems. By understanding how our jaws work, we can focus on relaxing various muscles to relieve pain. Hot pads to increase circulation or cold packs or anti-inflammatory medication to decrease pain and swelling are often

Lips Together, Teeth Apart, Tongue in Place

By repeating this phrase as a mantra we can heighten our awareness of the ideal posture for the mouth at rest.

used in conjunction with exercise to achieve optimal results.

We need to be conscious of our mouth position. The ideal position is one in which the teeth are a few millimeters apart, the tongue rests lightly at the junction of the upper teeth and gum tissue and the lips rest lightly together. The head should also be held in an upright, balanced but relaxed position.

We need to be aware if we habitually jut our chins forward or clench our teeth because we're angry, or bite down hard on pencils or pen caps while stressed at work, or engage in any other unconscious habits that place additional strain on our jaws. When times are tough, we may sustain a poker face and clench or tighten the muscles by holding our teeth tightly together. It is during such times that clenching during the daytime, and grinding and clenching during the night may occur. We need to pay attention to how we feel when we wake up. We need to ask ourselves these questions: Do my jaws ache? Do I have a headache? Do my teeth feel like they have had a workout and I have not even eaten breakfast?

Our teeth are designed to give us a lifetime of service. Teeth were *not* designed for grinding or clenching. The pressure on the enamel and dentin can cause premature wear and tear. Imagine if you were driving your car with the brakes on, the brake pads would wear out very quickly.

Each of us can use a technique called a "facial scan" to become more aware of the tension we may hold in our jaws or face.

A facial scan is performed by closing our eyes and asking ourselves:

- Are my skin and muscles tense, or relaxed?

- Are my teeth touching together lightly or tightly?

- Are my jaws hanging loosely with my lips together and teeth apart?

- Where is my tongue sitting? Is it behind my front teeth with the tip lightly touching my palate at the junction of the teeth and gum tissue? Or is it sitting on the floor of my mouth?

- Are my cheeks pulled into the sides where my teeth connect? Or do I chew my cheeks as an unconscious habit? (often this will create a white horizontal line on the inside of the cheek).

Breathing and Exercise

Once we become aware of poor habits involving our mouth, jaws or neck, we can take the necessary steps to restore a proper balance.

"Breathing may be considered the most important of all functions of the body, for, indeed, all the other functions depend on it."

- Yogi Ramacharaka, *The Hindu-Yogi Science of Breath*

Just as we are taught to massage our neck and shoulders, we can massage the muscles in our face, neck and jaws to provide relaxation.

We can also do certain exercises designed to relieve stress on our jaws, which can relieve headaches and other issues, such as clenching and grinding. These exercises should be done in conjunction with deep breathing. Yoga shows that deep, conscious breathing from the diaphragm allows for greater elasticity and stamina. Deep breathing helps to maximize the results of the exercises because we achieve a deeper release, faster. Deep breathing also helps us become more physically relaxed and emotionally centered as it expands the air pockets in the lungs, which brings about relaxation. By opening up our airways, more effective breathing delivers more oxygen to our bodies, a recognized remedy for relieving tension in our muscles. Such "breath therapy," combined with healing practices such as yoga, has often been found to alleviate and help manage headaches, chronic pain, hypertension, asthma, panic disorders and hyperventilation syndrome.

Think of your fingers as a warm iron carefully stroking and realigning the fibers of your muscles as if they were beautiful pieces of silk fabric; working out the nubbles (nodules) and aligning the threads.

Exercises That Can Be Done at Home

Undertake a facial scan (see page 57) prior to beginning these exercises and repeat once the exercises have been completed to see if your face looks or feels more relaxed.

During the exercises, try to maintain the ideal mouth position: *lips together, teeth apart, tongue in place.*

These exercises should be practiced on an ongoing basis to achieve their maximum effectiveness.

Intra-oral Exercises

The following exercises are used to find and release sensitive or sore trigger points in the following facial muscles: temporalis, masseter, lateral pterygoid and medial pterygoid. By checking the muscles daily, we can prevent storing tension in these areas.

1. Up, Out, Down and Back

(temporalis and masseter muscles)

Place your right index finger inside the right side of your mouth above the upper molar and parallel to your upper teeth between the teeth and cheek, and pull *upward and outward.*

Studies show that even light
clenching over time can cause
significant damage and
inflammation and lead
to muscle pain.

Now place your right thumb on the outside of the cheek. Using that thumb and the finger already inside your mouth, grip the muscle and stroke *down and back* toward the angle of the jaw.

Continue stroking the muscle *downward* until it is no longer tender and any knots or nodules are massaged out so that the muscle is smooth.

Repeat on the left side by placing your right thumb on the inside your mouth. Pull *upward and outward*. Using the index finger on the outside, grip the muscle and stroke *down and back* toward the angle of the jaw.

Continue stroking the muscle *downward* until it is no longer tender and any knots or nodules are massaged out so that the muscle is smooth.

If the muscles are very tight, they may not relax right away and repeated massage may be necessary.

2. Back and Up (lateral pterygoid)
Place your index finger on the biting surface of the last upper molar and roll this finger *back and up*. This can often produce tenderness.

Hold and gently press to release any tension. Once the muscle has no tension in it, you will feel how

Identifying Extra-oral
Exercise Points

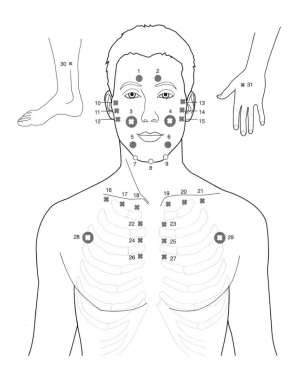

⊛ : massage the belly of these major muscles

● : use a light touch to "Feel the Pulse"

✸ : trigger points to massage

○ : points for "Jaw-ercise"

relaxed it can be. When repeated daily, this muscle will maintain a more relaxed tone. Repeat on the other side.

3. Down and Back (medial pterygoid)

With your index finger, feel the junction of the gum tissue and the lower back molar next to your tongue. Now stroke *down and back*. If tender, continue to stroke gently until no longer sore. Repeat on the opposite side.

Extra-oral Exercises

1. Touch and Massage

a. Touch and massage each of the three points in front of your ear (see points 10-15 on page 64). If the point or area is not tender in response to pressure, move on to the next point. If it is sore or tender, massage the point using deep breaths to release the tension. Increase the pressure while breathing in. Hold the spot while exhaling and feel the tension dissipate. Once the area is no longer tender to touch, move on to the next point.

b. Healthcare practitioners suggest that massaging the following points stimulates the lymphatic system, improves posture and enhances overall well-being.

Daytime low-level clenching
in healthy individuals may result
in more long-term fatigue and
muscle soreness than in those who
experience high-level grinding and
clenching for shorter durations.

Touch and massage the acupuncture point K27 (points 18 and 19), the major pectoralis muscles (points 28 and 29) and the other key trigger points (points 16, 17, 20-27, 30 and 31 on page 64) indicated on the diagram including the acupuncture points LI4 (large intestine 4) on the hand, and the Sp6 (spleen 6) on the ankle. If the point or area is not tender in response to pressure, move on to the next point. If it is sore or tender, massage the point using deep breaths to release the tension. Increase the pressure while breathing in. Hold the spot while exhaling and feel the tension dissipate. Once the area is no longer tender to touch, move on to the next point. As taught by health practitioners, tightness in the pectoralis muscles can pull the shoulders forward, altering posture and possibly contributing to head and jaw misalignment.

2. Clench and Release

Clench your teeth and use your middle finger to feel the belly (the center) of the jaw (masseter) muscle (see points 3 and 4 on page 64) pop out. Now unclench your teeth, but keep your finger in the same position and massage with small circular motions to release the tension.

Downward Jaw

This exercise releases stress
held in the jaw joint.

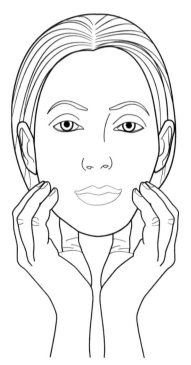

"Yoga's slow exercises provide
welcome relief to painful joints."

- Swami Saradananda, *Teach Yourself Yoga
for Health and Happiness*

3. Feel the Pulse

The pulse points are in two areas. These are indicated by points 1, 2 and 5, 6 of the diagram on page 64.

Touch lightly with your index, middle and third finger from both hands simultaneously and feel a pulse emerge. It can take 20 to 40 or more seconds to feel this light pulse. It releases and softens the external layer of skin that envelops the muscles and helps with facial tone.

4. Downward Jaw

With your teeth apart, secure both borders of your lower jaw with your index fingers and thumbs just above the angle of the jaw line and gently pull down and forward (See illustration on page 68). Hold for 30 seconds while feeling a gentle release.

5. "Jaw-ercise"

This is an excellent exercise for anyone with a limited range of mouth opening, hyperflexibility of muscles, headaches caused by teeth grinding or clenching or jaw instability.

Create a fist and hold it lightly under your lower jaw (see point 8 on page 64). Open the mouth with about two fingers' width between your front teeth

Ways to alleviate grinding and clenching:

- Reduce stress

- Apply ice or heat to sore jaw muscles

- Avoid eating hard foods like nuts and candies

- Drink plenty of water

- Get adequate sleep

- Learn stretching exercises to help restore a normal balance to the action of the muscles and joints on each side of the head

- Search out painful nodules, called trigger points, that can cause pain throughout the head and face

- Learn to relax your face and jaw muscles throughout the day

- Practice deep, intentional breathing as taught in yoga

- Practice "smile therapy"

- Repeat: **Lips together, teeth apart, tongue in place**

and press against your chin with your fist, creating light pressure, for 10 seconds. Now place your fist against the angle of your jaws and tense the jaw to match the light pressure being exerted by your fist. Hold for 10 seconds with the teeth apart. Repeat on the opposite side (see points 7 and 9 on page 64). Do this exercise for 30 seconds (10 seconds under the jaw, 10 seconds on the right side and 10 seconds on the left side) four times a day.

6. Smile Therapy

Never underestimate the importance of the simple act of smiling. Smile therapy is a natural therapeutic approach to rebalancing our emotions so that we reduce anxiety and stress, which can have many negative consequences including headaches and teeth grinding and clenching. It is based on research that shows that when we smile, our brain receives a signal that we are happy, pumping endorphins into our body. Endorphins reduce pain, enhance our immune system, and make us feel and look better. Just remembering to smile can do wonders in relieving stress on the mouth and entire body. Smile therapy can involve placing stickers or notes strategically on our computers, cell phones or mirrors to remind us to smile throughout the day.

4

SNORING AND SLEEP APNEA

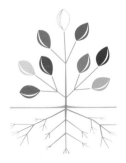

The soundness of our sleep directly impacts our wellness, our relationships and our ability to enjoy life.

A good night's sleep, like food and water, is a prerequisite for a healthy life.

Studies now confirm that when we breathe well we create the best conditions for health and well-being. Alternatively, when we don't breathe well, we become more susceptible to illnesses like high blood pressure and heart disease.

It is therefore not surprising that a temporary stoppage of breathing during sleep, also known as sleep apnea, can have dire consequences for our health. Researchers continue to add to our understanding of why sleep is so necessary to human and animal life. First, it helps repair damaged and worn tissue. More important, perhaps, is what it does for the brain. It not only appears to recharge it, but allows us to replay social interactions and carefully shade experiences with emotional color so that they are more understandable to us. It also allows us to sort and separate important facts from trivia and boosts our mental performance, learning and memory. In addition, sleep improves our ability to make novel connections among seemingly unrelated ideas. In other words, it sparks our creativity.

According to a 2009 survey by the National Sleep Foundation, only 28% of Americans get the recommended seven to eight hours of sleep–a drop of 10% since 2001. What's worse, losing one hour of sleep per night for a week is as detrimental to our health as going an entire night without sleep.

How to Get a Good Night's Sleep

- Establish and maintain a regular bedtime
- Start a nighttime routine
- Create a relaxing sleep environment
- Avoid eating two hours prior to bedtime
- Practice regular exercise routines
- Avoid caffeine, nicotine and alcohol prior to sleeping

Snoring

The sounds of snoring occur because there is an obstruction to the free flow of air through the passages at the back of the mouth and nose during sleep. This may be caused by something simple like our posture–sleeping on our backs–or congestion, alcohol intake, extra throat or nasal tissue, the position of our tongues, or abnormalities in the soft tissues of our throats. It can also be a major signal of sleep apnea. It is therefore important to find the cause of a snoring problem and identify the effects it may have on our health.

What Is Sleep Apnea?

Sleep apnea is a temporary stoppage in breathing during sleep. It is an all-too-common disorder thought to affect about 2 to 9 percent of women, 4 to 24 percent of men, and about 2 percent of children in North America, with the higher percentages among people between 50 and 59 years of age. And the number of people with sleep apnea continues to rise with the increase in obesity. Alarmingly, sleep apnea can reduce one's lifespan by as much as eight years. What's worse, it's

Signs of sleep apnea:

Do you snore?

Are you tired when you wake up?

Are you likely to doze off while sitting and reading? Watching TV? Riding in a car?

Snoring is a common cause of marital strife, causing some couples to seek out separate sleeping quarters–even houses. In the past, snoring was even considered proper grounds for divorce. It may come as little surprise, since the volume of an average snore can be measured between 60 and 90 decibels. At the low end, that's the equivalent to sleeping next to a dishwasher; at the upper end, it's like trying to sleep next to a lawn mower.

estimated that anywhere between 85 and 90 percent of sufferers go undiagnosed.

The most common symptom of sleep apnea is excessive snoring. Other symptoms include fitful sleep, excessive daytime sleepiness, memory changes, depression and irritability. In some patients it can even contribute to high blood pressure, heart failure, stroke and heart attack. It has also been linked to childhood issues, such as bedwetting, irritability and Attention Deficit Disorder (ADD)/Attention Deficit Hyperactivity Disorder (ADHD).

There are three main categories of apnea, but the most common, which is of increasing concern to the dental profession, is known as obstructive sleep apnea, or OSA. OSA is characterized by pauses in breathing during sleep caused by a physical block to the airflow. The muscles in the throat, mouth and tongue relax. They sag and narrow the airway, and the tongue slides to the back of the mouth creating a potentially deadly choke by blocking the windpipe and cutting off oxygen. The sleeper gasps for air, wakes up briefly and falls back to sleep in a cycle that repeats itself. Each episode lasts 10 seconds or

Consider these facts:

- Sleep apnea can reduce your lifespan by eight years

- 80% of sufferers go undiagnosed

- Sleep apnea takes a heavy toll on your cardiovascular system: 40% of stroke victims, 50% of people with hypertension and 40% of people with some form of myocardial condition have sleep apnea

- Without 25% REM sleep, your learning retention ability and even your creativity decrease

- 80% of those who have been diagnosed with ADD/ADHD have a sleep problem

- Sleep deprivation can cause depression, gastric reflux, a slow reaction time, weight gain and gout

- Sleep apnea decreases quality of life, making you tired, irritable, depressed and more prone to headaches

- Sleep apnea is linked to an increase in car accidents

- The sudden jerking of the body to reactivate breathing at night forces the gastric juices beyond the lower esophageal sphincter. This is one of the causes of gastroesophageal reflux disease (GERD) also known as acid reflux more and can occur from 5 times per hour to as often as 100 times or more per hour.

People with sleep apnea often don't get enough REM (rapid eye movement) sleep, the deep and restful stage of sleep that repeats about every 90 minutes during the night. They are thereby being robbed of sleep's most powerful restorative powers.

The Dentist's Role in Diagnosing and Treating Sleep Apnea

Some people have a genetic predisposition to develop sleep apnea and dentists can play a critical role in detecting additional risk factors. They can alert patients to enlarged tonsils or adenoids, which may obstruct the airway by forcing a person to breathe through the mouth rather than the nose. Excessive body weight may also result in extra tissue that can constrict the airway. Other predisposing factors include hypothyroidism, alcohol consumption, age (most common between ages 40 and 60) and gender (8:1 ratio male to female with severe apnea).

A large neck size, dark circles under the eyes or lips not fully closed can also alert dentists to possible

Breathing through the mouth
instead of the nose can decrease
oxygen intake by as much as 20%.

sleep disruptions. Underdeveloped arches on the top jawbone and the shape of the lower jawbone can also contribute to sleep apnea because they cause the tongue to sit lower in the mouth and create pressure on the airway at night. In short, throat obstruction or allergies can cause mouth breathing, which in turn creates a collapse of the upper arch and forces the tongue to sit lower in the mouth, putting pressure on the airway during sleep and possibly resulting in snoring and/or sleep apnea.

Dentists, along with other healthcare professionals, are conducting interesting studies into alternative ways to strengthen our upper airways and reduce or eliminate mild to moderate sleep apnea. They have found that exercising the muscles in the upper airways and the throat, for example, may help reduce the symptoms. One study showed that there is no sleep apnea among the Australian aboriginal tribes, whose members regularly play a long, hollow instrument called a didgeridoo. (Originally made only by hand from the eucalyptus tree, didgeridoos are now widely available in a variety of materials.) The researchers concluded that this was because the circular

Exercises for Snoring and Sleep Apnea

Our windpipes can range from being very weak tubes to very strong structures. A strong windpipe can support continual airflow and lead to fewer apneic episodes.

1. Place the tip of your tongue against the front of your palate and slide your tongue back and forth. Repeat this action throughout the day. The more the better! This simple exercise can strengthen your throat and help you sleep more restfully.

2. Exercising muscles in the upper airway may help improve symptoms of mild to moderate sleep apnea. One way these muscles can be strengthened is by playing a didgeridoo–an Australian aboriginal wind instrument. The circular breathing method required to generate the continuous droning sound produced by the instrument strengthens the windpipe.

breathing technique required to play the didgeridoo strengthens the windpipes of the players and consequently prevents collapse.

Beyond the CPAP Mask

Until relatively recently, the most common choice for treating sleep apnea, beyond weight loss, tonsil removal and perhaps some minor surgery of the nose or soft palate, was a CPAP mask. CPAP stands for continuous positive airway pressure. The mask is worn over the nose or nose and mouth during sleep, while compressed air is gently forced through the nose to keep the airway open. If properly calibrated, the CPAP mask ensures that the body receives proper airflow.

However, patient studies continue to show that far too many people fail to use their CPAP machine as indicated due to noise, size, discomfort and interference with romantic ambience. Fortunately, dentists can also recommend special bite plates and other oral appliances for the successful treatment of mild to moderate sleep apnea and snoring. These are used to keep the soft tissue from collapsing and

Screening Tool for Sleep-Disordered Breathing in Children

- Does your child snore?

- Does he/she sleep restlessly?

- Does he/she wet the bed?

- Is your child tired upon waking, and/or does your child have dark circles under his/her eyes?

- Does your child fall asleep or daydream during school?

- Does your child have behavioral problems?

- Is he/she irritable or aggressive?

- Has your child been diagnosed with ADD/ADHD?

- Do you ever hear your child stop breathing for 10 to 20 seconds at night, followed by choking or waking up?

interrupting normal breathing patterns by advancing the lower jaw. There are a wide variety of oral appliances available to help with sleep apnea. The most popular are adjustable to allow for structural changes to your mouth and jaw over time.

A dentist, working in conjunction with a sleep specialist, can also assess if structural changes may be helpful as a longer term solution. Orthodontics, restorative procedures and/or surgical corrections may help reposition the jaw, allowing better positioning of the tongue, maximizing airflow and reducing the number and severity of sleep apneic episodes.

If you have apnea or are at all concerned that you might, it is important to be tested. If mild to moderate sleep apnea is found, speak with a dentist about possible solutions to prevent serious health and lifestyle risks.

If sleep apnea is properly treated with a CPAP mask or oral appliance, long-term sufferers often report–even after only one night's sleep–that they feel like a million dollars!

5

ALIGNMENT AND THE MOUTH-BODY CONNECTION

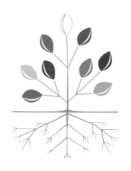

Dentistry combines with other health disciplines–including medicine, physiotherapy, chiropractic, osteopathy and naturopathy–to try to achieve overall harmony of the body.

Our head is delicately balanced on top of the spinal column by muscles in the jaws, neck, shoulders and back. Think of it another way: imagine that the head is a baseball balanced on top of a pencil with the help of a number of rubber bands. When the muscles are tense, they shorten. Now imagine shortening just one of these rubber bands. Some of the other bands would stretch, while some would shorten to accommodate for the shorter band and the baseball would be thrown off kilter. Similarly, when even a single jaw, neck or shoulder muscle becomes tense or shortened, all the other muscles are forced into overdrive just to keep the head balanced on the spinal column.

Balance, as taught by yoga, is about our ability to remain interconnected. We use considerably more energy to compensate when our balance is off and realigning becomes that much more difficult, painful and draining.

It's easy to see why reducing or eliminating shoulder aches, tension and tinnitus (ringing in the ears) may go beyond what happens in the dental chair. Although the source may be in the mouth, such pain often radiates to other areas. That's why dentistry is really about integrated care. It calls upon traditional and nontraditional healthcare professionals, as well as stress-release therapy, asking that each of us become more aware of the tension stored in our body.

With the adult head weighing an average of 10 pounds, it is easy to see how a forward posture of the head could be devastating to the entire neuromuscular system. When the neck is eight degrees forward, it creates a pull of 35 to 40 pounds of extra weight on the neck vertebrae and supporting muscles.

Establishing Harmony

Just as the health of our gums and teeth are intimately linked to the health of the rest of our body, a misalignment or collapse of the bite can also have a devastating impact on how the rest of our body functions. It can lead to dozens of problems, including headaches, neck and shoulder aches, ringing in the ears and sleep apnea.

The focus of dentistry is on the diagnosis and treatment of issues affecting the jaws, teeth and surrounding musculature. When our bite is off, the muscles in the jaws and face try to compensate for it, straining to bring our teeth closer together. These issues can often radiate beyond the head and neck, and this is where other healthcare practitioners can help balance the system.

The body can be perceived as being divided into three main structural zones: the head, the torso and the pelvis. These are connected by the spine. They are designed to stay in balance–the head, torso and pelvis should all be level with one another. To maintain normal balance, our body compensates for injury in one area by distributing stress to other areas.

Planes of the Face

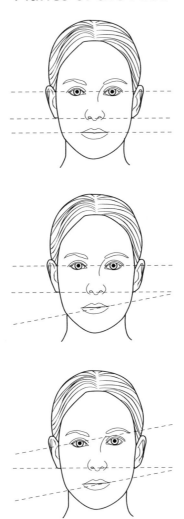

Balance can be negatively affected by problems that travel down the body, which include bite and temporomandibular joint (TMJ) problems. These are called "descending" problems. Balance can also be adversely affected by problems that travel up the body, such as uneven leg length, which are called "ascending" problems. Healthcare practitioners who specialize in body structure report that these situations are seldom isolated–if someone has an ascending problem, chances are that they also have a descending problem and vice versa. It has been found that best results are most often achieved by taking into account the function of the nervous system and balancing the body as a whole.

Some Associated Problems

Think of the head as also having its own three planes–through the eyes, ears and mouth. Ideally these three planes strive to be horizontal and parallel to each other. However, sometimes the teeth in the upper jaw don't run parallel to the eyes or ears. They may slant (or cant) upward on one side. The problem can be further complicated because one or more teeth may be twisted, or partly rotated. If the teeth are out of sync with the

Our jaw joint is the only joint in our body that we cannot live without.

other two planes, the bite isn't perfectly parallel and the descending structures have to cushion the strain, resulting in pressure on the surrounding muscles and joints.

The TMJ may also be a source of problems. The muscular system that controls the jaws and keeps the head propped up is extraordinarily complex. For example, the muscles that allow the jaws to open for biting and swallowing–which they do several hundred times a day–are all interconnected in the neck. The power muscles that allow us to chew and that keep the jaws from falling open extend from the jaws upward through the cheeks into the forehead and behind the ears. The brain is programmed to subconsciously hold the jaws at a position where the teeth are close to fitting together, but not in actual contact.

If everything is just right and the jaws are not moving, most of these muscles are said to be at rest, or barely working to maintain the ideal position–*lips together, teeth apart, tongue in place.* However, if the bite is unstable from poorly aligned teeth or even a missing tooth, the muscles have to work a lot harder just to bring the teeth

Our tongue may not be something we want to see, but this powerful muscle is a hard-working "multi-tasker." Our tongue helps us talk, eat, chew, swallow, even fight germs. The tongue houses the majority of our taste buds, which help us savor our food. Our tongue also helps us articulate our words, sing our songs, and because it can twist, stretch and turn, it enables us to clean our mouths of sticky food or food debris.

together, and become strained. And when the muscles are under constant strain, they become painful. A domino effect results as other muscles may also become involved.

The Tongue as a Bully Muscle

When our tongue is placed properly in position inside our mouth, it helps balance the lower jaw position from the inside. It also helps to mold and hold our teeth and arch in position. The ideal position for the tongue is for its tip to be resting where the gum tissue meets the inside of the two upper front teeth.

We can verify whether our tongue is sitting in its ideal position by repeating the phrase or mantra: *lips together, teeth apart, tongue in place.* Now check to see if the tongue is in position, behind the upper teeth, touching the junction of the tooth and gum tissue.

If the tongue is not in the ideal position, its sheer force through the action of swallowing can actually tip and move teeth. This means that if for some reason one is forced to breathe through the mouth, perhaps because of allergies or obstructive breathing, the tongue moves farther back and

You can tell if your mouth
is in the ideal position
by repeating this mantra:

Lips together, teeth apart, tongue in place.

Lips together, teeth apart, tongue in place.

Lips together, teeth apart, tongue in place.

Lips together, teeth apart, tongue in place.

Lips together, teeth apart, tongue in place.

Lips together, teeth apart, tongue in place.

Lips together, teeth apart, tongue in place.

Lips together, teeth apart, tongue in place.

down to make room. Over time the position of the tongue behind the lower front teeth causes the upper arch to narrow in the mouth. When the tongue is sitting low in the mouth we often see the formation of a double chin which, surprisingly, frequently has nothing to do with aging, weight gain or hereditary factors.

Fortunately, there are ways today to modify the internal space in our mouths so that the tongue can regain its proper space and resting position. When dealing with children, dentists assess when genetics, environmental or neuromuscular factors are interfering with ideal tooth and jaw formation. Telltale signs may be narrow arches, crowded teeth, high palate and incorrectly developed jaws. With children we can help the bone grow in a controlled direction, rather than remodel the bone later in life. Through special appliances we can help reshape the jaws as they grow so that there is space for all the teeth, allowing room for proper tongue position.

6

THE POWER OF THE FOOD WE CHEW

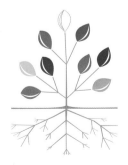

Making good choices about what we eat and drink is important for overall health, as well as for optimal dental health.

Unhealthy food choices promote tooth decay, tooth erosion and excessive wear of tooth enamel. Nutritional eating, on the other hand, sustains firm and healthy gum tissue, which protects our heart from excessive bacteria buildup and prevents the transmission of bacteria from the mouth to the rest of our body.

Our diet has changed more since the beginning of the 20th century than at any other point in human history and not for the better. While industrialization has reduced the body's need for a high-calorie diet, new technologies have revamped the food supply by introducing thousands of processed foods. So many of today's foods are rife with extra fat, sugar and chemicals—preservatives, emulsifiers, food coloring and the like that are extracted and often processed in combination with other food additives that aren't even listed on the label!

Good nutrition requires eating a variety of food groups. There are some basic rules of nutrition to follow: pick fresh, unprocessed food; consider organic options with fewer pesticides and toxins; and choose monounsaturated oils and complex carbohydrates. To do this we need to become familiar with the ingredients in the foods we choose and their characteristics. We also need to be aware of the value of various nutrients, vitamins and minerals, and consciously include them in our diet, even if this means taking supplements (as advised by a qualified healthcare professional). There are also foods that we ought to eat less of, such as those that can cause excess acidity, or should avoid altogether, such as those with refined sugars, refined flours and additives.

The foods we choose to nourish
and sustain us play a defining
role in our wellness.

Our Food, Our Health

Nutrition is the process by which organisms obtain energy in the form of food for growth, repair and maintenance. Today, however, our nutrition levels are being threatened by various factors. We often select too many unhealthy foods and not enough nutrient-dense foods, a practice that directly affects our nutrition levels and the way our bodies function. There are some foods that might seem to be healthier choices, but should still be avoided. For example, hard granola bars may require a bite force that can exceed human bite strength and therefore may result in fractured or broken teeth. We also store and cook food in ways that decrease its nutritional benefits. For example, we may start with fresh fruits and vegetables, but, through cooking they lose much of their nutritional value. Raw fruits and vegetables provide us with the most nutrients and essential enzymes.

Such habits have a cumulative effect on our mouths and bodies. We are a culture lacking essential nutrients and suffering from dietary imbalances caused by overeating, choosing the

Of the leading causes of death today, five are linked to poor diet: heart disease, stroke, diabetes, liver disease and some cancers.

wrong foods and not exercising enough. Many in our population are mineral deficient and lack the enzymes found in raw fruits and vegetables, which allow us to use nutrients to create energy and stamina. Without the ability to draw energy from our food, our immune systems are less effective in protecting our health, leaving us vulnerable to disease and chronic degenerative conditions. Vitamin D taken with magnesium, for example, helps with the absorption of calcium. Vitamin D can be produced by our body when we are exposed to sunlight in the summer months. However, winter sunlight is not sufficient for our body to metabolize vitamin D from sunshine. We may require a supplement if our levels are low, which can be determined through a blood test. As we age, our ability to produce our own enzymes diminishes and the quality of the foods we choose, and our ability to chew well, become even more important.

Nutritional Pioneer

Weston Price, a dentist and nutritional pioneer working in the 1920s and 1930s, was among the first modern researchers to study the connections between the ancestral diet and health–specifically

In the 1920s, a typical grocery store stocked 800 items while today even a small supermarket offers 10,000 goods–and 17,000 new products show up every year!

the impact of diet on the teeth and gums. His findings were published in his 1939 book *Nutrition and Physical Degeneration*.

Price studied primitive tribes in places like Switzerland, Alaska, Tahiti, Samoa and Kenya. He found that many of the plagues of modern civilization, from headaches to heart disease, can be traced directly to a modern diet. He also found that those who ate a traditional diet weren't nearly as susceptible to tooth decay or periodontal disease. However, when native peoples suddenly changed their diets to include refined sugar and flour, Price noted a remarkable difference, not just in their health, but in their physical appearance. Due to the decreased need for chewing to break down processed foods, for example, the dental arches of subsequent generations became narrower, causing teeth to crowd.

Price's conclusions? No one diet is ideal for everyone. Optimal health requires the consumption of nutrient-dense whole foods and we can achieve optimum health by matching the traditional diets of our ancestors—which may have been primarily game, seafood, vegetation, dairy or any combination thereof.

Saliva is a protective gatekeeper and performs many functions. It:

- Helps you start digesting food before it even reaches the stomach

- Mixes with food to enable easier swallowing

- Contains a factor called histatins that accelerates wound closure of oral cells and facilitates healing

- Spreads molecules to the taste buds on the tongue so you can tell whether something is salty, sour, sweet, spicy, or, in some instances, dangerous to your health

- Is a good indicator of your overall health (by measuring its pH, see page 123)

- Helps lubricate the teeth, tongue and surrounding tissues

- Contains antibacterials that help wash away food particles and bacteria from around the teeth

Importance of Nutrition to the Oral Cavity

Over the decades evidence has mounted that poor food choices particularly affect our gums and teeth. The unique characteristics of the soft tissues of the mouth make them more sensitive to nutrition than other parts of the body. Nutritional deficiencies and toxicities, therefore, are often first noticeable in the oral cavity.

Our mouth and the way we eat also play a part in how much we get out of our food. Our digestive processes begin in the oral cavity. We initiate the process by biting and chewing to break our food into pieces that can be swallowed. If we eat under stress and too fast, we don't get as much value out of what we consume. When eating slowly, we allow time for the digestive enzyme amylase to be excreted into the saliva and begin to break down our food. The rule of thumb is to chew each bite 30 times prior to swallowing. By paying attention to chewing, a small, but important movement, we create less work for our digestive systems and acquire more nutrients.

Q: If you opened your lunch tomorrow and found a sandwich, a carrot and a cookie, in what order would you eat them?

A: Sandwich, cookie, carrot– because you don't want refined sugar to be the last food you eat, since it can begin to decay the teeth quickly. Foods like carrots and celery sticks clean your teeth after you eat.

The Damaging Effects of Eating Sugar

Undoubtedly our biggest dietary sin is the consumption of sugar. It wreaks havoc on our bodies, particularly our mouths. When combined with saliva and the bacteria in our mouths, it becomes the primary cause of tooth decay and contributes to gum disease. The problem is that sugar and bacteria are a formidable combination. Bacteria (plaque) feeds on the sugar. The end product is acid, which starts dissolving the tooth enamel and may eventually create holes or cavities.

Knowing that we cannot eliminate our intake of sugar altogether, we need to control the bacteria through proper oral hygiene and the removal of food remnants from our mouths as soon as possible. Surprisingly, bacteria are unable to differentiate between natural and processed sugars. Common culprits in tooth decay are dried fruits, which have high concentrations of naturally occurring sugars. The stickiness of dried fruits causes them to adhere to the recesses in and around the teeth where they cannot be easily rinsed off. This results in sugars spending more time in the mouth and can cause a great deal of

The following added sugars are typically found in food products:

- Granulated table, brown, corn, raw, turbinado, invert and powdered sugar
- Honey
- Maple syrup
- Molasses
- Glucose
- Levulose
- Lactose
- Dextrin
- Sucrose
- Mannitol
- Sorbitol
- Malt
- High fructose corn syrup
- Fructose
- Maltose
- Concentrated fruit juice
- Dextrose
- Isomalt*
- Stevia*
- Xylitol*

* Note: Some of these sugars, such as sugar from the herb stevia, Isomalt and xylitol, are considered a wiser choice. Stevia has been shown to stabilize blood sugar levels and not contribute to tooth decay. 100% xylitol in chewing gum or mints slows bacterial growth in the mouth, helping prevent decay.

damage. The problem is made worse for people with dry mouth syndrome, as they have limited saliva to aid in removing sugars from the teeth, and they can experience even greater rates of decay. If we can't brush after a meal containing sugar and other refined foods, we can help clean our teeth by eating fibrous foods, like raw apples and carrots, aged cheese, chewing pure xylitol gum and, happily, even eating a piece of dark chocolate will also work to raise the saliva pH toward an alkaline environment in which tooth decay is minimized.

From a nutrition viewpoint, sugar is also empty calories. It is too often consumed in place of protein, good fats, fiber, and vitamin and mineral-rich foods, giving us a sweet taste without nutritional value. Even worse, refined sugar actually requires considerable quantities of vitamins and minerals to metabolize, thus drawing these nutrients from where they can benefit the body.

Sugar also has a negative effect on our immune system. Yeast thrives on sugar and a diet high in starches and sugar can lead to Candida—a serious fungal overgrowth in the body—particularly for

Baby Bottle Tooth Decay
(also called nursing caries)

Prolonged contact with the simple sugars of fermentable carbohydrates in liquids such as milk, formula, juice and even breast milk can lead to rapid tooth decay in infants and young children. This often results from a baby falling asleep while nursing a bottle or breastfeeding: the liquid pools around the teeth and the bacteria in the baby's mouth turn the sugar into acid.

those with compromised immune systems. This can lead to a series of conditions, such as pain, depression, fatigue and body dysfunction. Sugar also neutralizes the positive effects of essential fatty acids and lowers white blood cell activity. One teaspoon of refined white sugar has been said to decrease the effectiveness of the immune system for 45 minutes or more.

Glycemic Index and Glycemic Load

Along with our sugar addiction, we are a culture obsessed with fats and carbohydrates. We examine every label to see if an item is "fat-free," often not realizing that the missing fat or carbohydrate has been replaced with refined sugar.

Many believe that all carbohydrates are the same. They are not. Different carbohydrates behave quite differently and trigger different reactions when ingested. Most foods, whether processed or natural, contain carbohydrates, which the body breaks down into simple sugars to be absorbed into the bloodstream. This is the major source of energy for the body.

Glycemic Load
High: 20+, Medium: 11-19, Low: 10 or less

	Approximate GL per Average Serving
Non-starchy vegetables (peas, carrots, beans, etc.)	1-3
French fries (1/2 cup)	24
Baked potato	26
Boiled potato	14
Orange	5
Apple	6
Banana	15
Raisins (1/2 cup)	30
White rice (1 cup)	23
Brown rice (1 cup)	18
White bread (1 slice)	10
Whole wheat bread (1 slice)	9
White bagel	25
Spaghetti (1 cup, white, boiled)	22
Spaghetti (1 cup, whole wheat, boiled)	15
Packaged cereals (1 cup)	12-22
Chocolate bar	20
Peanuts	1
Soft drinks	15-23
Orange juice	13
Skim milk	4

When we eat carbohydrates, the rate at which it turns into sugar is measured by the food's "glycemic index" (GI). The carbohydrate content of the food is measured by its "glycemic load" (GL).

Some foods, like carrots, have a high glycemic index, but a low glycemic load. This means that, although the carbohydrates in a carrot are quickly absorbed into the bloodstream, there is little carbohydrate content to begin with and so it is unlikely to cause a negative response.

Most "fast foods" are low in both fiber and nutrients. They are "quick fix" foods that provide instant gratification and usually have both a high glycemic index and a high glycemic load. These foods satisfy us temporarily because they raise our blood sugar quickly and it stays elevated for a period of time, but then we experience an energy "crash" and feel hungry again. These foods are also more refined, with higher sugar levels, and can lead to tooth decay. On the other hand, foods with a low glycemic index and a low glycemic load are "sustaining foods." They are metabolized more slowly and make us feel full because they produce only small fluctuations in our blood glucose

pH stands for 'potential hydrogen'. It is a measurement of the acidity of water when the hydroxyl OH molecules and the hydrogen H+ molecules balance each other out.

and insulin levels. Not only are such foods key to sustainable weight loss and a healthy body, but they are low in sugar and lead to improved dental health.

In general, it is important to minimize our intake of refined or processed "bad" carbohydrates and instead choose natural "good" carbohydrates—such as vegetables—which are nutrient-dense and high in fiber.

Acidity

We are increasingly learning how unbalanced acidity in the body can be detrimental to wellness. Acidity is measured by the pH scale—a chemical yardstick that indicates whether a substance is acidic or alkaline. The pH scale ranges from 0 to 14, with a reading between 0 and 6.9 indicating a decreasingly acidic environment and a reading between 7.1 and 14 one that is increasingly alkaline. A reading of 7 is considered neutral. These numbers are measured on a rapidly increasing scale.

An acidic environment in the mouth can cause a great deal of damage to the teeth in the form of tooth decay and excessive enamel erosion.

Raw broccoli, cauliflower and carrots should be part of a healthy diet. The more times you chew these vegetables, the more nutrients you extract from them. The process of cooking often destroys vital elements in such foods.

Ongoing high acidity in the mouth may be the result of poor food and beverage choices or the chronic regurgitation of stomach acids caused by acid reflux or bulimia. As a result of its destructive force, dentists are becoming increasingly aware of the importance of monitoring the pH level of saliva.

Many other conditions and ailments have also been associated with overly acidic environments. Signs that our cells are too acidic may include low energy, headaches, depression and mouth ulcers. There are also numerous negative health effects associated with environments that are too alkaline. The goal is to achieve balance, and the commonly accepted healthy pH level of saliva is between 6.4 and 7.4.

Luckily our body has the capability to balance itself at a neutral pH provided we supply it with the right ingredients. By choosing fresh, nutrient-dense, unprocessed foods we give our body the tools it needs to create and maintain a balanced system that optimizes our health and well-being. Uncooked, organic fruits and vegetables are the backbone of life. They have the

Swish and Swallow

After eating, if you're unable to brush, it's always good to take a drink and do the swish and swallow technique.

Ten-Minute Rule

90% of damage in your mouth occurs 10 minutes after you've finished eating. Therefore it's essential to clean away the sugar residue after eating sweets. This can be done by eating something as simple as a piece of old cheddar cheese or dark chocolate, since they are good for neutralizing acidity.

Two-Hour Rule

After an acidic meal or after drinking an acidic beverage, wait one to two hours before brushing your teeth. The acid weakens the tooth structure if you brush immediately. A two-hour delay allows the teeth to re-mineralize. However, you can minimize acidity by eating alkalizing foods or increasing your water intake.

highest concentration of enzymes that feed our metabolism by supplying energy to our body and truly are the best medicine. Calcium is also helpful to decrease the body's acidity.

Processed foods and beverages like alcohol, sports drinks and soft drinks change the normal pH balance of the body and interfere with its use of alkaline minerals, such as sodium, calcium, magnesium and potassium. Sports drinks in particular can create a dangerously high acidic environment that can be very damaging to our teeth. From a dental perspective, when we bathe our mouth with an acidic drink, our teeth begin to decalcify and become more prone to erosion and mechanical breakdown. It has been said that it takes the body five hours to return to a more neutral pH after consuming an acidic beverage.

A system that is too acidic can also inhibit the immune system and make us more susceptible to chronic diseases. In contrast, a nutrient-rich diet results in healthier tissues in the body. A healthier, balanced environment reduces the risk of disease, maintains good health and reduces tooth decay.

Research shows that people who consume a high-glycemic (high sugar) breakfast consume 80% more calories throughout the day.

We need to remember that we also bring acidity into our cells when we are emotionally or physically stressed: our hearts beat faster, our muscles tense, our metabolism increases and so does our acidity level! Meditation and regular exercise are both methods that can help decrease the stress levels that increase acidity and also activate the lymph system that removes acidic waste products.

We can test the pH level of our saliva using pH strips. These strips can usually be purchased at a pharmacy or health food store and ideally provide measurements in increments of 0.2. Note that saliva should not be tested within two hours of eating or drinking in order to ensure an accurate reading. Swish your saliva around in your mouth and swallow. Then repeat to ensure the saliva is fresh and clean. Now, place some saliva on the paper. A pH test that shows a highly alkaline or acidic reading may be an indicator of a possible health problem that one might want to discuss with a doctor. If caught early, a further decline in health may be avoided.

What to Eat: A Basic Checklist

- Natural, fresh, whole foods

- A variety of fruits and vegetables daily

- A variety of grains daily, especially whole grains

- White meats and fish (but be aware that high levels of mercury and other toxins may be present in large ocean fish, including tuna, swordfish and shark)

- Unsaturated fats such as olive oil, olives, nuts, natural peanut butter, almonds and avocados

- Foods that are low in saturated fat and cholesterol, and moderate in total fat

- Foods and beverages that have moderate or low sugar levels

- Foods with less salt

- Complex carbohydrates because they take more time to digest

- About eight glasses of water a day for digestion and metabolism

- Look at the food on your plate. A variety of color indicates that you will be consuming a variety of nutrients

Making Good Choices

In many ways, choosing what to eat has never been more complicated. At one point there was a tide of "carbophobia" and we were advised to load our plates with meats and fats. A few years later carbohydrates were back in fashion and fats were the no-no. This type of scientific back-and-forth has contributed to what best-selling author Michael Pollan has called our "national eating disorder." His advice? "Eat food. Not too much. Mostly plants."–a dietary credo that is simple and makes sense.

One thing that most healthcare practitioners certainly do agree on is that we need to eliminate as many processed foods from our diet as possible.

7

THE POWER OF BEING POSITIVE

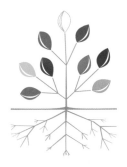

When we have a healthy and attractive mouth, we feel better about ourselves; we tend to smile more and in doing so we can actually improve our overall health and well-being!

More than a century ago, Charles Darwin predicted that science would one day unravel the physiological mechanisms of emotion; in other words, the connection between the mind, the body and the spirit.

Certainly the idea that our minds and bodies are closely intertwined is not new. In fact, it's a fundamental precept in many Eastern and alternative theories of medicine. But the idea that our minds can influence our bodies found new credibility within Western medicine in the late 1970s when a PhD student named Candace Pert, working in a lab at the Johns Hopkins University School of Medicine, made a startling discovery—a breakthrough that would provide a road map to explain how feelings and behavior impact health and disease.

According to Pert, emotions stem from electrochemical signals that affect the chemistry and electricity of every cell in the body. Her theory, in a nutshell, is that the interaction of the immune, nervous and endocrine systems is essentially a network in which these systems communicate with one another. Pert did pioneering research on chemical links between the brain and the rest of the body, and demonstrated that emotions could be reduced to chemicals called neuropeptides. She also discovered the opiate receptors in our brain, leading the way to the discovery of endorphins, the brain's natural painkillers.

Pert's discovery, and subsequent book, *Molecules of Emotion: The Science Behind Mind-Body Medicine*, is a major contribution to an exploding branch of science called psychoneuroimmunology, or PNI, an interdisciplinary study that combines psychology, neuroscience, immunology, pharmacology and molecular biology, among other sciences. Pert's discovery has given credence to the notion that our body is a reflection of our mind and that we each have the potential to help heal ourselves by stimulating the release of endorphins through the management of our thought processes. In other words, we can achieve a healthier state through the power of positive thinking.

Yoga teaches us about connectivity—we cannot separate what goes on in our bodies from what goes on in our minds.

What Is Positive Thinking?

At its core, positive thinking is an attitude that fosters thoughts, words and images conducive to success. It's an attitude that can assist in bringing happiness, health and successful outcomes to each and every situation. We can almost tell if people are thinking in a positive way by the look on their faces–they carry a natural smile. Our positive attitude also comes from how we set ourselves up for life's disappointments. If we insist on defining idealized expectations, we will be profoundly disappointed when these are not fulfilled. But if we work on changing our expectations to aspirations, our disappointment diminishes. Instead of forcing our desires into becoming our experience, we allow life to progress as it will. This helps us rebound into a positive frame of mind more quickly when the occasional and inevitable adversity is encountered.

The Nun Study

An exhaustive research project known as *The Nun Study* showed that nuns who had a more positive attitude outlived their more pessimistic

Both inner and outer peace
begin with a smile.

counterparts by a hefty margin. Beginning in the early 1990s, Alzheimer's researcher and gerontologist David Snowdon studied 678 nuns who were at least 75 years old at the School of Sisters of Notre Dame, an American order of Catholic nuns. The nuns gave Snowdon unprecedented access to their medical and personal records, many dating back to the days when they were new to their vocation. Snowdon scored their short autobiographies for positive emotional content. He found that a distinct pattern emerged: those with the most positive emotions lived on average 6.9 years longer (to an average of 93.5 years) than those who scored lower on the positivity scale. Perhaps the more optimistic attitude was summed up best by one sister who, on her 106th birthday, declared: "I've had so much fun, I think I'll stick around another year."

Don't Forget to Smile

Smiling relieves stress in the mouth. Research also shows that when we smile, our brain receives a signal that we are happy and endorphins pump into our body. Endorphins reduce pain,

"Your Honour deigns to smile?
Your smile is fair as flow'rs.
Thus spake the wise Ocunama:
A smile conquers all, and defies
ev'ry trouble. Pearls may be
won by smiling;
Smiles can open the portals
of Paradise.
The perfume of the Gods,
the fountain of Life,
Thus spake the wise Ocunama:
A smile conquers all,
defies ev'ry trouble."

Excerpt from *Madame Butterfly*, L. Illica & G. Giacosa;
R.H. Elkin/Giacomo Puccini

enhance our immune system and make us feel and look better.

Research by French physiologist Israel Waynbaum demonstrates that when we frown, we suppress our immune system by increasing stress and blocking energy. Waynbaum showed that the facial muscles we use to smile, on the other hand, can trigger endorphins, as well as immune-boosting, killer T-cells. When we smile we also lower stress hormones like cortisol and adrenalin, while stabilizing blood pressure, relaxing muscles, improving respiration and speeding up healing. A healthy and beautiful smile also helps us to build a positive self image.

It's almost impossible to smile on the outside without feeling better on the inside. Though we often think happiness precedes a smile, the opposite is also true. Studies show that *even when we force ourselves to smile*, natural endorphins are released into our systems that elevate our mood. The next time you are having a bad day, try smiling and see if that helps turn things around. The effect may even be enhanced if you go to the mirror. Researchers have shown that seeing a

When we smile we actually lower stress hormones, like cortisol and adrenalin, while stabilizing blood pressure, relaxing muscles, improving respiration and speeding up healing.

smile will activate our smiling muscles and we'll feel happier.

Laughter

Laughter has also been proven to be downright healthy, and our mouth is the chamber through which our laughter is set free. Like smiling, laughter creates a mood in which positive emotions are put to work for us and those around us to strengthen the immune system, stimulate circulation, decrease blood pressure and increase the body's natural painkillers–endorphins.

In 1979, the editor of *Saturday Review*, Norman Cousins, published a story about the power of laughter. He had been given six months to live due to a painful, degenerative disease of the spine. Desperate to find some relief, he discovered that 10 minutes of laughter gave him two hours of pain-free sleep. After several months, the restorative benefits of the sleep, combined with his ongoing medical treatment, enabled Cousins to walk out of the hospital well again.

His story baffled scientists. Although many scorned his findings, his subsequent book,

"Laughter is a tranquilizer
with no side effects."

- Arnold H. Glasgow

Anatomy of an Illness, inspired a number of research projects. Ten years later *The Journal of the American Medical Association* published a vindicating article: "Laugh If This Is a Joke." In the article a Swedish medical researcher named Lars Ljungdahl concluded that sustained laughter "can increase the quality of life for patients with chronic problems and that laughter has an immediate symptom-relieving effect."

Another proponent of the power of laughter, Dr. Madan Kataria, founded a school called Laughter Yoga. Today the American School of Laughter Yoga is the oldest and largest provider of Laughter Yoga education in North America. Inspired by and still affiliated with Dr. Kataria's school, clubs teach ways to create, strengthen and sustain personal and group laughter with the belief that this will lead to enhanced physical and mental health, improved social skills, a higher resilience to stress, greater emotional intelligence and increased overall cognitive ability.

The Benefits of Meditation

Meditation is one of the Five Principles of Yoga

Yoga practices and meditations teach us how to release the stresses that cause pain not only physically but also emotionally.

and has been shown to have beneficial effects. It is a stress-reduction technique that is highly advocated to release tension in the face; alleviating grinding and clenching and the pain we often experience as a result.

Meditation is a type of mindfulness or awareness that involves purposeful breathing while focusing the mind on present thoughts and actions.

Transcendental meditation is taught worldwide and involves sitting comfortably with eyes closed and muscles relaxed while silently repeating a mantra (usually a single syllable) for a period of about 20 minutes. Whether the mantra is spoken or silent, the energy still resonates from and within the mouth.

Herbert Benson, a professor at Harvard Medical School, was one of the first scientists to research meditation and how it can be used to trigger a "relaxation response." His published work illustrates how meditation can result in many health benefits, including the reduction of stress and its many negative impacts such as high blood pressure, heart disease and chronic pain.

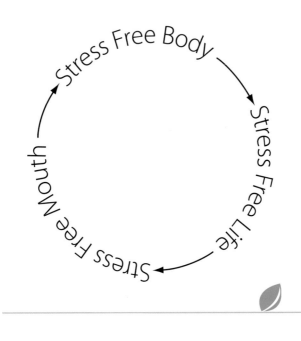

Jon Kabat-Zinn, a professor of medicine emeritus at the University of Massachusetts Medical School, has also done extensive research on the effects mindful meditation has on healing. He has shown that meditation is a stress-reduction technique that can positively affect the brain, immune system and other areas of the body, reducing pain, promoting healing and enhancing well-being.

The Choice Is Ours

Having and sustaining a healthy mouth and beautiful smile helps us build a positive attitude about ourselves.

Researchers do not yet know the exact extent to which psychological factors create or prolong a disease. We need to be careful in making sweeping statements, such as "Happy people don't get sick," but there is certainly a good deal of evidence that positive emotional factors enhance healing and that negative thinking can predispose an individual to chronic diseases.

Our smile is our best
natural vitamin.

As the old saying goes, "Laughter is the best medicine." Laughter has been shown to increase oxygen intake, lower blood pressure and release endorphins. Ancient wisdom and modern research has also shown that proper deep-breathing techniques can ward off disease by making people less susceptible to viruses, lowering blood pressure and decreasing cholesterol levels.

Best of all, the decision to smile or not, laugh or resist, or face the day with an optimistic or negative attitude is entirely within our control.

8

FEELING EMPOWERED AND FULL OF POTENTIAL

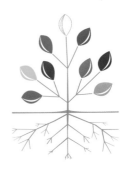

Over the years, shifting and crowding of teeth can occur in our mouth.

It's only at rare moments that we stop and think, *Oh, my teeth have changed*. Some of us notice, while others do not see a change, just as we may or may not pay attention to how our body shifts and changes.

However, what we see in front of us when we look in the mirror has the potential to make us feel empowered. At a time when North American men and women are spending thousands of dollars on face and neck creams, a corrected smile can be a far more effective way to bring about a youthful transformation.

The high level of sensitivity in our mouths resonates throughout our body—from a structural to an emotional and energetic level. But it all begins with the mouth. Confident and radiant smiles truly are symbols of hope. They allow our communication to come from a clean and beautiful place; when we smile, we open a window to the soul.

Today's new knowledge and technology allows us to set the stage for the next several decades of our life. This step may be taken at any age–whenever we decide the time is right for us.

Undoubtedly it's been a journey to come to the point where we have now arrived, just as the study of yoga is a lifelong journey of working our way toward a more enlightened place. Think of it this way: at first the *ABCs* become words. Then words become sentences. And sentences become paragraphs. Eventually, there's an understanding of the bigger picture and with that comes growth. Looking at these patterns, the various integrated parts that have come together over the years, allows us to approach dentistry with a sense of gestalt–a feeling of confidence that the pieces of the puzzle are finally coming together!

9

YOGA FOR
THE MOUTH

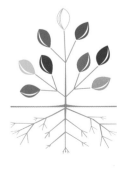

Many believe yoga is simply an exercise. Yes, yoga teaches exercises–deep conscious breathing, as well as stretches for better posture, balance and energy.

But yoga is also a science and philosophy about the integration of body and mind. Yoga literally means "to yoke" in Sanskrit, which refers to the "yoking together" or unifying of body and mind, with the intent of realizing our connectedness and wholeness.

How does this relate to looking after our mouth? The wholistic principles and practices of yoga, which strive for overall mental and physical health, can be applied to caring for our mouths to achieve optimal oral health, which is an integral part of overall health.

Science today is teaching us that the mouth is not a closed system, but one connected to the rest of our body. The health of our mouth is affected by the health of our body and vice versa. Gum disease is a bacterial infection in the mouth and the same bacteria can travel through the bloodstream and put our entire health at risk. When the health of our mouth deteriorates through decay or gum disease, it may put our general health in jeopardy, particularly if we have additional risk factors. By making this critical connection between what goes on in our mouth and the rest of our body, we are taking the first step toward optimal health.

Yoga teaches us about being mindful to maintain and improve our bodies over a lifetime. By being mindful, educated and aware of our choices, we take responsibility for our well-being. And it's each person's responsibility to be the guardian and protector of his or her own body.

Yoga also shows us how small, conscious movements can bring about long-term results. When we begin yoga, we are reminded to "go at our own pace."

Being Mindful of the Power of Our Choices

Yoga is about being mindful. By being mindful of the choices we make regarding our mouths—the hardness of the foods we eat, how we brush, how we chew, even how we hold the posture in our jaws, lips and tongue—we have the power to bring about and sustain good dental health.

Think about it for a moment. Our mouth is the most sensitive place in our body, detecting every particle that we place into it. Even how we chew, with small mindful movements, enhances the digestive process and our ability to extract essential nutrients.

Making Small Movements and Slow Shifts

Yoga is also about the importance of small, conscious movements to strengthen our emotional and physical well-being. A minimally invasive approach to dentistry is the same. Using new technology, gentle orthodontic forces allow the bone to remodel itself slowly over time and regain better balance for teeth, muscle and soft tissue. Through these small movements and slow shifts, we are able to remodel our mouths at any age.

Yoga reminds us to continually embrace the breath of life. Breathing is more than a respiratory exchange of carbon dioxide and oxygen; it is our very life force. The importance of deep, proper, rhythmic breathing for health, energy and well-being is not confined to yoga alone.

Practicing Proper, Deep, Rhythmic Breathing

Deep, rhythmic breathing can work wonders in strengthening weak airways. If we can strengthen and expand the airway leading into our mouth, we can achieve better overall health and even extend the length of our lives. Proper nasal breathing, especially when we exercise, also brings an increased oxygen supply into our bodies.

Through a combination of deep breathing and meditative techniques, many yoga followers have found freedom from physical pain and emotional suffering—factors that can have a direct effect on the tension people carry in their bodies and their mouths. Studies have proved again and again what Eastern health traditions have known for centuries—when we breathe consciously, we create optimal conditions for health and well-being. By breathing well, we create space for our minds and bodies to relax; we allow compassion for ourselves and increase opportunities for healing.

Strengthening Our Mouth's Inner Core

Just as yoga focuses on strengthening our "inner core," dentistry looks to strengthen our mouth's

Yoga emphasizes the value of posture, balance and flexibility. When we align our bodies correctly, we strengthen our inner core both physically and emotionally.

inner core. The inner core of our mouth is comprised of our jawbones and arches (the U-shaped curvature of the teeth–ideally wide versus narrow). The misalignment of our mouth's inner core can have a domino effect throughout the body with serious repercussions on our overall health.

Luckily, it is now possible to straighten teeth, better align arches and widen smiles at any age. The goal is to create symmetry in the mouth, make the bite more comfortable and allow teeth to fit together more precisely. The resulting smile adds better balance to the whole face.

We can also strengthen the inner core of our mouth by being more conscious of our mouth posture. We can learn to do this by repeating the mantra: *Lips together, teeth apart, tongue in place.*

Practicing Respect, Acceptance and Acknowledgment

Our mouth is a visual display of our happiness. This is why it is so important that we care and show respect for oral health. Our mental attitude also affects our body, both inside and out. It shines through our faces and smiles when we smile,

Yoga asks that we continually expand and stretch our muscles. By stretching and working our muscles to firm and strengthen them, we release muscle tension and create a fuller range of motion–and better alignment–in our bodies.

laugh, sing or speak positively about one another.

There is much research that reinforces the importance of our attitude, positive or negative, on our overall physical health. When we say kind words to each other, we greet the world in a positive manner, showing each other respect and acceptance. When we smile, we radiate our happiness. Endorphins from our brains actually make us feel happier; smiling makes us look younger and even live longer!

Learning to Expand and Stretch

Yoga has demonstrated the benefits of relieving muscle pain through stretching. Similarly, it is important to stretch and expand the muscles in and around the mouth, which, if stressed, can lead to grinding and clenching, and may result in headaches, excessive wear and erosion of teeth, gum recession, clicking and cracking in the jaw joint, and tight jaw muscles. Dentists can provide specialized dental appliances, jaw and mouth exercises, and trigger-point massage therapies for the mouth that help expand tight muscles over time. By applying this technology and these

Yoga instructs us about the
relationship we have with
the rest of the world. We are
all interconnected. Yoga greets
us with "Namaste"–an attitude
of acknowledgment,
acceptance and respect.

techniques, it is possible to reduce and even relieve the debilitating tension in the mouth that can radiate to other parts of our body.

Yoga Exercises for the Mouth

In addition to the exercises found on pages 57-71, the following exercises decrease tension, protect the teeth from the heavy stresses of grinding or clenching, and enhance good breathing. They also allow for a more youthful and relaxed face. These exercises utilize all the major auxiliary and interconnected muscles and do not involve using your hands. They are good for activating these muscles to strengthen and create firmer facial tone—a good addition to wellness and a fountain of youth!

Relaxed Face

Close your eyes, relax and imagine a point between the eyes. Hold for one minute. This is good for stress release.

Tongue Stretch

Stick out your tongue and stretch it as far as it can go. Hold for 60 seconds. Then slowly retract the tongue over the roof of your mouth in a forward and back motion. Repeat the forward and back motion 20

"Yogic lifestyle is one of compassionate self-discipline based on the ideals of simple living and high thinking."

-Swami Saradananda, *Teach Yourself Yoga for Health and Happiness*

times. Complete four times daily. Practiced regularly, this helps develop a tighter musculature, which may help strengthen the windpipe and can help lessen the severity of sleep apnea.

Smiling Fish Face

Smile while pursing your lips and hold for 10 seconds. Repeat three times. This works the muscles around the mouth and can help reduce the appearance of aging.

Baby Bird

Swallow while pressing the tip of the tongue to the roof of your mouth. Then, with the tip of your tongue still pressing on the roof of your mouth, tilt your head up and slightly to the left and swallow. Repeat to the right. Complete the cycle five times. This exercise helps tighten the internal muscles, which can prevent the formation of jowls and may also help prevent sleep apnea.

Facial Stretch

Open your eyes wide and puff out your cheeks as much as you can. Hold for 10 seconds. Repeat three times. This alleviates grinding and clenching.

A CLOSING WORD FROM THE AUTHOR

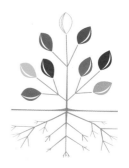

"We shall never know the good a simple smile can do...."

This book has looked at both the form and function of the mouth from many angles. We have explored its role in our well-being from the view of sustaining healthy gum and bone tissue. We have looked at how grinding, clenching, and jaw and tongue position influence headaches, our physical structure and the quality of sleep. The chapter "The Power of the Food We Chew" discussed the importance of proper nutrition with respect to acidity, the hardness of foods and pressures they exert on our teeth, and the impact of sugar. In "The Power of Being Positive" we examined the impact of our mouth on the power of words, speech and communication, both silent and spoken. I continue to be amazed at how the mouth–as the instrument for delivery of a healthy and confident smile–can encourage in us greater self-esteem.

Throughout this book we have used yoga as an analogy, as we have learned in preventative dentistry that our patients need to own and understand their dental health. We also have learned that light gentle forces move teeth with less resistance. Alignment in the mouth is reflected elsewhere in the body. And yoga exercises for the mouth and face can be our fountain of youth.

My intent in this book is to create awareness about the importance of the mouth and our role in sustaining this gift, and to understand and undertake more than the daily maintenance of brushing and flossing. When this awareness occurs we can fully honor and care for the gift we have been given.

I have seen so many unhealthy mouths over the years, at many levels of decay, unhealthy bone support and excessive wear. I feel sad knowing how much more pristine and healthy these mouths could be if the patients could start again using the knowledge we have today. My hope is that my patients and readers will be able to understand and embrace the information shared in this book and will treasure their mouth even more than they have in the past.

What surprises me again and again is how, when teeth become aligned or even a single front tooth is modified, the face and smile–and subsequently the head posture–will often appear more relaxed and balanced, resulting in a wider smile. Wider smiles create facial volume. Widening the scaffolding allows the skin to drape properly, creating a fuller, more balanced and youthful face.

As the past ten years has brought photography into our daily work, we are now able to capture oral images within seconds to share chair-side. This allows us to co-discover and share findings with patients, and together design a treatment plan that is both comfortable for them and allows them to go at their own pace. Not everything needs to be done at once and with an awareness of available options a plan can be put in place that prevents further deterioration. Knowledge is power.

You never know better health until you get there! I challenge you to help yourself or a loved one to maximize the quality of the life that we have been gifted. A beautiful smile is possible for everyone regardless of age, and I encourage you to explore with your dental professional what it takes to turn a dream into a reality.

Your smile radiates and reflects your inner beauty and is your best natural vitamin, a true gateway to a healthier you!

ACKNOWLEDGMENTS

This book has been a passion of mine for the past few years. It represents a compilation of much that I have learned and experienced throughout my dental career.

There are many people who have contributed to my education that I would like to thank. The first are my parents for their unconditional love and for always believing in me. The second is my sister Anita Rachlis, who has always held the highest standards in education and who has taught me, through her constant striving for excellence and her love for the medical profession, that education is unending.

Thank you to my children, Jeffrey and Caitlin, for your patience, understanding and support. And thanks to all my friends and extended family including Val Rachlis, Shelley Black, Charlie Hodgekinson, Greg Mahon, Stefanie Hill, Caron Rambeau, Bonnie Newman and Harold Newman for all your support and listening.

My greatest teachers have been my team members. The dentists that I work with—Urusa Ansari, Bernie Gryfe and Leyla Emami—are wonderful people with great skills and warm hearts. The rest of my team—Rosie, Caron, Stevka, Karen, Sharon, Terri, Sandy, Ljiljana, Lana, Margaret, Sandra, Jessica, Dejana, Patricia, Nick, Maria, Natasha, Fran, Norma, Maryam, Ling, Samantha, Lucy, Kinga, Monika, Katherine, Miki and Hayla—many of whom have been with me for over 20 years, have shown me how it is possible to be better each day than the day before, as they continually focus on the quality of care they provide to the people who visit us. I thank you all.

To my patients: thank you for your trust and for allowing me the opportunity to work with you.

The thousands of hours spent in continuing education have involved many mentors who have helped me synthesize a greater understanding and a way of practice reflected in Wellness Based Dentistry™. Some of these mentors include the Pankey Institute, The Group at Cox, Wilson Southam, Bud Ham, Doug Young, Avrom King, Carol McCall, Cathy and John Jameson, Dr. Jim Carlson, Dr. Bob Walker and Dr. Kaye

McArthur, Dr. Ed Spiegel, Dr. Barry Glassman, Dr. Jean Pascal, Dr. John Kois, the AACD and the IAOMT.

I would also like to thank the following people who graciously volunteered their time to ensure the text was clearly presented and understood so that readers could receive the most value possible from the book: Dr. Kat Nobrega-Porter, Dr. Linda Finn, Dr.Tim Jaegar, Dr. Colin Shapiro, Dr. Peter Birek, Emily Ridout and Christine Russell. Thanks also to Karen Bone for helping with the title and to Barbara Stoneham for your energy and commitment in creating my photo for the book jacket.

A very special thank you to Rosemary and Jay Whiteside and Dr. Chuck Marino for your invaluable help and guidance.

Thank you to Dan Sullivan of The Strategic Coach Inc. for the sharing of a larger world.

And thank you to my Book Project Manager and Editor, Susan Hart, who has shown so much patience and enthusiasm in making this book become a model on how we can appreciate and care for our mouths every waking moment.

BIBLIOGRAPHY

Much of the content in this book represents an accumulation of the author's knowledge gained through dental school, continuing education and travels to foreign countries to learn about their dental practices and beliefs. Many of the specific sources used in the development of the text are listed below as tools for those wishing to learn more about a specific topic. Additional information can also be found at: www.YOURMOUTHthegatewaytoahealthieryou.com.

Section 1: The Power of the Mouth

AACD, *Survey of American Public*. American Academy of Cosmetic Dentistry 2004.

Bodane C, Brownson K, *The Growing Acceptance of Complementary and Alternative Medicine*, Health Care Manager 2002; Volume 20 Issue 3. Pages 11-21.

Evans CA, D.D.S., M.P.H., Kleinman DV, D.D.S.,MSc.D., *The Surgeon General's Report on America's Oral Health: Opportunities for the Dental Profession*, The Journal of the American Dental Association 2000; Volume 131, Issue 12, Pages 1721-1728.

Fortier S, *Community Leadership: Inside and Out*. Zip Lines: The Voice for Adventure Education 1999; Volume 38, Pages 43-46.

Goldstein RE, D.D.S., *Change Your Smile*, 3rd Edition, Quintessence Publishing, 1997.

Mitsis FJ, *Hippocrates in the golden age: his life, his work and his contributions to dentistry*, The Journal of the American College of Dentists Spring 1991; Volume 58, Issue 1, Pages 26-30.

Price WA, *Nutrition and Physical Degeneration: A Comparison of Primitive and Modern Diets and Their Effects*, Paul B. Hoeber Inc., Medical Book Department of Harper & Brothers, 1939.

Pritchett P, *Hard Optimism*, McGraw-Hill, 2007.

Roizen MF, M.D., *RealAge: Are You as Young as You Can Be?*, HarperCollins Publishers, 2001.

Vukovic A, Bajsman A, Zukic S, Secic S, *Cosmetic dentistry in ancient times - a short review*, Bulletin of the International Association for Paleodontology 2009; Volume 3, Issue 2, Pages 9-13.

Zoumalan RA, Larrabee WF Jr., *Anatomic considerations in the aging face*, Facial Plastic Surgery 2011; Volume 27, Issue 1, Pages 16-22.

Section 2: The Whole Body Connection

Axelsson P, Paulartder J, Lindhe J, *Relationship between smoking and dental status in 35-, 50-, 65-, and 75-year-old individuals*, Journal of Clinical Periodontology 1998; Volume 25, Issue 5, Pages 297-305.

Bosy A, *Oral malador: philosophical and practical aspects*, The Journal of the Canadian Dental Association March 1997; Volume 63, Issue 3, Pages 196-201.

Brown TT, Cruz ED, Brown SS, *The effect of dental care on cardiovascular disease outcomes: an application of instrumental variables in the presence of heterogeneity and self-selection*, Journal of Health Economics September 29, 2010. (Epub ahead of print)

Canadian Dental Hygienists Association Position Statements, Review of the Oral Disease-Systemic Disease Link. Part II: Preterm Low Birth Weight Babies, Respiratory Disease, January-February 2007; Volume 41, Issue 1, Pages 8-21.

Chapple, ILC, *Potential Mechanisms Underpinning the Nutritional Modulation of Periodontal Inflammation*, The Journal of the American Dental Association 2009; Volume 140, Pages 178-184.

Elter JR, White BA, Gaynes BN, Bader JD, *Relationship of Clinical Depression to Periodontal Treatment Outcome*, Journal of Periodontology 2002; Volume 73, Pages 441-449.

Fisher MA, Taylor GW, Papapanou PN, Rahman M, Debanne SM, *Clinical and Serologic Markers of Periodontal Infection and Chronic Kidney Disease*, Journal of Periodontology 2008; Volume 79, Pages 1670-1678.

Friedewald VE, Kornman K, Beck JD, Genco R et al., *The American Journal of Cardiology and Journal of Periodontology Editors' Consensus: Periodontitis and Atherosclerotic Cardiovascular Disease*, The American Journal of Cardiology 2009; Volume 80, Issue 7, Pages 1021-1032.

Gazolla CM, Ribeiro A, Moysés MR, Oliveira LAM, Pereira LJ, Sallum AW, *Evaluation of the Incidence of Preterm Low Birth Weight in Patients Undergoing Periodontal Therapy*, Journal of Periodontology 2007; Volume 78, Issue 5, Pages 842-848.

Greenstein G, Lamster L, *Changing Periodontal Paradigms: Therapeutic Implications*, The International Journal of Periodontics & Restorative Dentistry 2000; Volume 20, Pages 337-357.

Johnson GK, Hill M, *Cigarette Smoking and the Periodontal Patient*, Journal of Periodontology 2004; Volume 75, Pages 196-209.

Kibayashi M, Tanaka M, Nishida N, Kuboniwa M, Kataoka K, Nagata H, Nakayama K, Morimoto K, Shizukuishi S, *Longitudinal Study of the Association Between Smoking as a Periodontitis Risk and Salivary Biomarkers Related to Periodontitis*, Journal of Periodontology 2007; Volume 78, Issue 5, Pages 859-867.

Lin D, Moss K, Beck JD, Hefti A, Offenbacher S, *Persistently High Levels of Periodontal Pathogens Associated with Preterm Pregnancy Outcome*, Journal of Periodontology 2007; Volume 78, Pages 833-841.

Mesley B, The *Interactions Between Physicians and Dentists in Managing the Care of Patients with Diabetes Melitus*, Journal of the American Dental Association 2008, Volume 139, Pages 1-7.

Nogueira-Filho G, Tenenbaum HC, *So Why Call It the Oral-Systemic Health Connection?* The Journal of the Canadian Dental Association 2011; Volume 77, Page 36.

Offenbacher S, Beck JD, Moss K, Mendoza L et al., *Results From the Periodontitis and Vascular Events (PAVE) Study: A Pilot Multicentered, Randomized, Controlled Trial to Study Effects of Periodontal Therapy in a Secondary Prevention Model of Cardiovascular Disease*, Journal of Periodontology 2009; Volume 80, Issue 2, Pages 190-201.

Reddy MS, *Reaching a better understanding of non-oral disease and the implication of periodontal infections*, Journal of Periodontology 2000; Volume 44, Issue 1, Pages 9-14.

Rose LF, Steinberg BJ, Minsk L, *The Relationship Between Periodontal Disease and Systemic Conditions*, Compendium Continuing Education Dent 2000; Volume 21, Pages 870-878.

Rosenberg M, ed. *Bad Breath: Research Perspectives*. Tel Aviv, Israel: Ramot Publishing, Tel Aviv University, 1995; Pages 46-50, 87-89.

Tanner A, Kent R, Van Dyke T, *Clinical and Other Risk Indicators for Early Periodontitis in Adults*, Journal of Periodontology 2005; Volume 76, Pages 573-581.

Xiong X, Buekens P, Fraser W, Beck J, Offenbacher S. *Periodontal disease and adverse pregnancy outcomes: a systematic review*, BJOG: An International Journal of Obstetrics & Gynaecology 2006; Volume 113, Issue 2, Pages 135-143.

Section 3: Grinding, Clenching and Headaches

Carlsson GE, Magnusson T, *Management of Temporomandibular Disorders in the General Dental Practice*, Quintessence Publishing Co., Inc., 1999.

Davies C, *The Trigger Point Therapy Workbook: Your Self-Treatment Guide For Pain Relief*, New Harbinger Publications, 2001.

Dawson PE, *New Definition for Relating Occlusion to Varying Conditions of the Temporomandibular Joint*, Journal of Prosthetic Dentistry 1995; Volume 74, Issue 6, Pages 619-627.

Ehsani S, Alsulaimani M, Thie N, *Why do dentists need to know about myofascial pain?*, Journal of the Canadian Dental Association 2009; Volume 75, Issue 2, Pages 109-112.

Farhi D, *The Breathing Book: Good Health and Vitality Through Essential Breath Work*, Owl Books, 1996.

Gessel AH, D.D.S, Alderman MM, D.D.S., *Management of Myofascial Pain Dysfunction Syndrome of the Temporomandibular Joint by Tension Control Training*, Psychosomatics, 1971; Volume 12, Pages 302-309.

Howat JMP, *Chiropractic: Anatomy and Physiology of Sacro Occipital Technique, Headington,* Oxford: Cranial Communication Systems Ltd., 1999, Pages 133-157.

Josell SD, *Habits affecting dental and maxillofacial growth and development,* Dental Clinics of North America 1995; Volume 39, Issue 4, Pages 851-860.

Kurita H, Kurashina K, Kotani A, *Clinical effect of full coverage occlusal splint therapy for specific temporomandibular disorder conditions and symptoms,* Journal of Prosthetic Dentistry 1997; Volume 78, Issue 5, Pages 506-510.

Page DC, D.D.S., *The orthodontic shift toward functional jaw orthopedics,* The Functional Orthodontist 2000; Volume 17, Issue 4, Pages 14-17.

Page DC, D.D.S., *Your Jaws Your Life,* SmilePage™ Publishing, 2003.

Sheikholeslam A, Holmgren K, Riise C, *A clinical and electromyographic study of the long-term effects of an occlusal splint on the temporal and masseter muscles in patients with functional disorders and nocturnal bruxism,* Journal of Oral Rehabilitation 1986; Volume 13, Issue 2, Pages 137-145.

Travell JG, M.D. and Simons DG, M.D., *Myofascial Pain and Dysfunction: The Trigger Point Manual,* Waverly Press Inc., 1983.

Yogi Ramacharaka, *The Hindu-Yogi Science of Breath,* CreateSpace, 2009.

Section 4: Snoring and Sleep Apnea

Bader G, Kampe T, Tagdae T, Karlsson S, Blomquist M, *Descriptive Physiological Data on a Sleep Bruxism Population,* Sleep 1997; Volume 20, Pages 982-990.

Bader G, Kampe T, Tagdac T, *Body Movement During Sleep in Subjects with Long-Standing Bruxing Behavior*, International Journal of Prosthodontics 2000; Volume 13, Issue 4, Pages 327-333.

Chan J, Edman JC, Koltai PJ, *Obstructive sleep apnea in children*, American Family Physician March 2004; Volume 69, Issue 5, Pages 1147-1154.

Cheshire K, Engleman H, Deary I, Shapiro C, Douglas NJ, *Factors impairing daytime performance in patients with sleep apnea/hypopnea syndrome*, Archives of Internal Medicine 1992; Volume 152, Issue 3. Pages 538-541.

Gray LP, *Results of 310 cases of rapid maxillary expansion selected for medical reasons*, The Journal of Laryngology & Otology 1975; Volume 89, Issue 6, Pages 601-614.

Gregory-Head B, Curtis DA, *Erosion Caused By Gastroesophageal Reflux: Diagnostic Considerations*, Journal of Prosthodontics 1997; Volume 6, Issue 4, Pages 278-285.

Guimarães KC, Drager LF, Genta PR, Marcondes BF, Lorenzi-Filho G, *Effects of Oropharyngeal Exercises on Patients with Moderate Obstructive Sleep Apnea Syndrome*, American Journal of Respiratory and Critical Care Medicine 2009; Volume 179, Issue 10, Pages 962-966.

Hang WM, *Obstructive Sleep Apnea: Dentistry's Unique Role in Longevity Enhancement*, Journal of the American Orthodontic Society 2007; Volume 7, Issue 2, Pages 28-32.

Holmgren K, Sheikholeslam A, Riise C, *Effect of a Full-Arch Maxillary Occlusal Splint On Parafunctional Activity During Sleep in Patients with Nocturnal Bruxism and Signs and Symptoms of Craniomandibular Disorders*, Journal of Prosthetic Dentistry 1993; Volume 69, Issue 3, Pages 293-297.

Lavigne GJ, Goulet J, Zuconni M, Morisson F, Lobbezoo F, *Sleep disorders and the dental patient: An overview, Oral Surgery, Oral Medicine, Oral Pathology,* Oral Radiology, and Endodontology 1999; Volume 88, Issue 3, Pages 257-272.

Macaluso GM, Guerra P, Di Giovanni G, Boselli M, Parrino L, and Terzano MG, *Sleep Bruxism is a Disorder Related to Periodic Arousals During Sleep,* Journal of Dental Research 1998; Volume 77, Page 565.

National Sleep Foundation, 2009 Sleep in America™ Poll: Highlights and Key Findings. Washington, DC: National Sleep Foundation, 2009.

O'Connor GT, M.D., MS, Lind BK, MS, Lee ET, Ph.D., Nieto J, M.D., Ph.D., Redline S, M.D., MPH, Samet JM, M.D., MS, Boland LL, MPH, Walsleben, Ph.D., Foster GL, MA, *Variation in Symptoms of Sleep-Disordered Breathing with Race and Ethnicity: The Sleep Heart Health Study,* Sleep 2003; Volume 26, Issue 1, Pages 74-79.

Page DC, D.D.S., *Your Jaws Your Life,* SmilePage™ Publishing, 2003.

Puhan MA, Suarez A, Lo Cascio C, Zahn A, Heitz M, Braendli O, *Didgeridoo playing as alternative treatment for obstructive sleep apnoea syndrome: randomised controlled trial,* British Medical Journal (BMJ) 2006; Volume 332, Issue 7536, Pages 266-270.

Selvaratnam P, Niere KP, Zuluaga MI, *Headache, Orofacial Pain and Bruxism: Diagnosis and multidisciplinary approaches to management,* Churchill Livingstone, 2009.

Sheikholeslam A, Holmgren K, Riise C, A *clinical and electromyographic study of the long-term effects of an occlusal splint on the temporal and masseter muscles in patients with functional disorders and nocturnal bruxism,* Journal of Oral Rehabilitation 1986; Volume 13, Issue 2, Pages 137-145.

Sjoholm TT, Lowe AA, Miyamoto K, Fleetham JA, Ryan CF, *Sleep bruxism in patients with sleep-disordered breathing*, Archives of Oral Biology 2000; Volume 45, Issue 10, Pages 889-896.

Thie N, Kimos P, Lavigne G, Major P, *Sleep structure, bruxism and headache*. In Selvaratnam P, Niere K, & Zuluaga M (eds.), *Headache, Orofacial Pain and Bruxism: Diagnosis and multidisciplinary approaches to management*, Churchill Livingstone Elsevier, 2009.

Young T, Palta M, Dempsey J, Skatrud J, Weber S, Badr S, *The occurrence of sleep-disordered breathing among middle-aged adults*, The New England Journal of Medicine April 1993; Volume 328, Issue 17, Pages 1230-1235.

http://www.surgeryencyclopedia.com/Pa-St/Snoring-Surgery.html

Section 5: Alignment and the Mouth-Body Connection

Davies C, *The Trigger Point Therapy Workbook: Your Self-Treatment Guide For Pain Relief*, New Harbinger Publications, 2001.

Dickerson WG, Thomas NR, *Accurately Transferring the Horizontal and Sagittal Relations*, LVI Visions 2006; Pages 17-25.

Ekfeldt A, Karlsson S, *Changes of Masticatory Movement Characteristics After Prosthodontic Rehabilitation of Individuals with Extensive Wear*, International Journal of Prosthodontics 1996; Volume 9, Issue 6, Pages 539-546.

Fonder AC, *The Dental Physician*, Medical Dental Arts. 2nd Revised Ed., 1985.

Bibliography

Garry JF, *Early iatrogenic orofacial muscle, skeletal and TMJ dysfunction*, In Diseases of the Temporomandibular Apparatus, D Morgan, House. Hall, Vamas. C.V. Mosby, St. Louis, 1982, Pages 35-69.

Gelb H, *The Optimum Temporomandibular Joint Condyle Position in Clinical Practice*, The International Journal of Periodontics & Restorative Dentistry 1985; Volume 5, Issue 4, Pages 34-61.

Howat JMP, *Chiropractic: Anatomy and Physiology of Sacro Occipital Technique*, Headington, Oxford: Cranial Communication Systems Ltd., 1999, Pages 133-157, 181-186.

Jankelson RR, *Neuromuscular Dental Diagnosis and Treatment*, Ishiyaku EuroAmerica Inc. 2nd Ed. 2005; Pages 1-12, 33-51.

Josell SD, *Habits affecting dental and maxillofacial growth and development*, Dental Clinics of North America 1995; Volume 39, Issue 4, Pages 851-860.

Magnusson T, Egermark I, Carlsson E, *A prospective investigation over two decades on signs and symptoms of temporomandibular disorders and associated variables*. A final summary, Acta Odontologica Scandinavica 2005; Volume 63, Issue 2, Pages 99-109.

McNeill C, *Management of Temporomandibular Disorders: Concepts and Controversies*, Journal of Prosthetic Dentistry 1997; Volume 77, Issue 5, Pages 510-522.

Mongini F, *Remodeling of the Mandibular Condyle in the Adult and its Relationship to the Condition of the Dental Arches*, Acta Anatomica 1972; Volume 82, Issue 3, Pages 437-453.

Page DC, D.D.S., *The orthodontic shift toward functional jaw orthopedics*, The Functional Orthodontist 2000;

Volume 17, Issue 4, Pages 14-17.

Page DC, D.D.S., *Your Jaws Your Life*, SmilePage™ Publishing, 2003.

Roth G, *The Matrix Repatterning Program for Pain Relief: Self-Treatment for Musculoskeletal Pain*, New Harbinger Publications, 2005.

Section 6: The Power of the Food We Chew

Attin T, Weiss K, Becker K, Buchalla W, Wiegand A, *Impact of modified acidic soft drinks on enamel erosion*, Oral Diseases 2005; Volume 11, Issue 1, Pages 7-12.

Auad S, Moynihan P, *Diet and Dental Erosion*, Quintessence International 2007; Volume 38, Issue 2, Pages 130-133.

Bezanis R, *pH Madness*, Neff/Harry Publishing, 2010.

Bland JS, Levin B, Costarella L, Liska D, Lukaczer D, Schiltz B, Schmidt M, Lerman R, Jones D, *Clinical Nutrition: A Functional Approach,* Institute of Functional Medicine, 2nd Ed., 2004.

Davis RE, Marshall TA, Qian F, Warren JJ, Wefel JS, *In Vitro Protection Against Dental Erosion Afforded by Commercially Available Calcium-Fortified 100 Percent Juices*, The Journal of the American Dental Association 2007; Volume 138, Issue 12, Pages 1593-1598.

de Almeida PDV, Grégio AMT, Machado MÂN, de Lima AAS, Azevedo LR, *Saliva Composition and Functions: A Comprehensive Review*, The Journal of Contemporary Dental Practice 2008; Volume 9, Issue 3, Pages 72-80.

Duffy W, *The Sugar Blues*, Warner Books Inc., 1976.

Elliott SS, Keim NL, Stern JS, Teff K, Havel PJ, *Fructose, weight gain, and the insulin resistance syndrome*, American

Journal of Clinical Nutrition 2002; Volume 76, Issue 5, Pages 911-922.

Hoza Farlow C, D.C., *Food Additives: A Shopper's Guide to What's Safe and What's Not*, KISS for Health Publishing, 2007.

Larsen M, Nyvad B, *Enamel Erosion by Some Soft Drinks and Orange Juices Relative to Their pH, Buffering Effect and Contents of Calcium Phosphate*, Caries Research 1999; Volume 33, Pages 81-87.

Mayanagi G, Kimura M, Nukaya S, Hirata H, Sakamoto M, Benno Y, Shimauchi H, *Probiotic Effects of Orally Administered Lactobacillus Salivarius WB21-Containing Tablets on Periodontopathic Bacteria: A Double-Blinded, Placebo-Controlled, Randomized Clinical Trial*, Journal of Clinical Periodontology 2009; Volume 36, Pages 506-513.

Nutrition for Docs: Using Nutritional Supplements in Clinical Practice. A Practical, Evidence-based Approach: Part I - Developing a Core Regime, and Part II, [Lecture at Dalla Lana School of Public Health Sciences, Family & Community Medicine University of Toronto.] April 17-18, May 29-30, 2010.

Price WA, D.D.S., *Nutrition and Physical Degeneration: A Comparison of Primitive and Modern Diets and Their Effects*, Harper & Brothers, 1939.

Pollan M, *In Defense of Food*, Penguin Group, 2008.

Sears B, M.D., *The Anti-Inflammation Zone*, HarperCollins Publishers, 2005.

von Fraunhofer JA, Rogers MM, *Dissolution of dental enamel in soft drinks*, General Dentistry 2004; Volume 52, Issue 4, Pages 308-312.

Wongkhantee S, Patanapiradej V, Maneenut C, Tantbirojn D, *Effect of acidic food and drinks on surface hardness of enamel, dentine, and tooth-coloured filling materials*, Journal of Dentistry 2006; Volume 34, Issue 3, Pages 214-220.

Young RO, Ph.D., Redford-Young S, *The Ph Miracle: Balance Your Diet, Reclaim Your Health*, Grand Central Publishing, 2010.

Section 7: The Power of Being Positive

Benson H, Stark M, *Timeless Healing: The Power and Biology of Belief*, New York: Scribner, 1996.

Cousins N, A*natomy of an Illness as Perceived by the Patient: Reflections on Healing*, New York: W. W. Norton & Company, 1979.

Danner DD, Snowdon DA, Friesen WV, *Positive emotions in early life and longevity: Findings from the nun study*, Journal of Personality and Social Psychology May 2001; Volume 80, Issue 5, Pages 804-813.

Darwin C, *The expression of the emotions in man and animals*, London: John Murray, 1872.

Kabat-Zinn J, Ph.D., *Full Catastrophe Living, Using the Wisdom of Your Body and Mind to Face Stress, Pain, and Illness*, Bantam Dell, 1990.

Kataria M, *Laugh For No Reason*, Madhuri International, 1999.

Ljungdahl L, *Laugh If This Is a Joke*, The Journal of the American Medical Association 1989; Volume 261, Issue 4, Page 558.

Locker D, Clarke M, Payne B, *Self-perceived Oral Health Status, Psychological Well-being, and Life Satisfaction in an Older Adult Population*, Journal of Dental Research 2000; Volume 79, Issue 4, Pages 970-975.

Myss C, Ph.D., *Anatomy of the Spirit, The Seven Stages of Power and Healing*, Crown Publishers Inc., 1996.

Pert CB, *Molecules of Emotion: The Science Behind Mind-Body Medicine*, Scribner, 1999.

Pritchett P, *Hard Optimism*, McGraw-Hill, 2007.

Shapiro D, *The Body Mind Workbook, Exploring How The Mind & The Body Work Together*, Element Books Inc., 1990.

Strack F, Martin LL, and Stepper S, *Inhibiting and Facilitating Conditions of the Human Smile: A Non-Obtrusive Test of the Facial Feedback Hypothesis*, Journal of Personality and Social Psychology 2008; Volume 54, Pages 768-777.

Waynbaum I, *La Physionomie humaine, son mécanisme et son rôle social*, Paris 1907.

Section 9: Yoga for the Mouth

Deepak C, Simon D, *The Seven Spiritual Laws of Yoga: A Practical Guide to Healing Body, Mind, and Spirit*, John Wiley & Sons, Inc., 2004.

Devi NJ, *The Secret Power of Yoga*, Three Rivers Press, 2007.

Farhi D, *The Breathing Book: Good Health and Vitality Through Essential Breath Work*, Owl Books, 1996.

Scott J, *Ashtanga Yoga*, Three Rivers Press, 2001.

Rama, Swami, *Exercises for Joints & Glands: Simple Movements to Enhance Your Well-Being*, 2nd Edition, Himalayan Institute Press, 2007.

Swami Saradananda, *Teach Yourself Yoga for Health and Happiness*, The McGraw-Hill Companies, Inc., 2007.

http://www.time.com/time/photogallery/0,29307,1683326_1484590,00.html

INDEX

Page locators shown in italics indicate an illustration.

10:00 – walk to D. (bring alterations? Boots?)
10:30 – Mani & Pedi →
11:00 – Bank – ask SRT USD
12:30 – shopping – coffee – fruit
1:00 – lunch
1:30 – travel name
2:00 – groom, shower, tan
2:30 –

3:30 – travel
4 hair